WELLNESS MADE SIMPLE

How to

KEEP CANCER & OTHER DISEASES AT BAY

Connie Boucher, LMT

You can purchase additional copies of this book at supersimplewellness.com
AromaTools.com

ISBN NUMBER: 978-1-4276-4733-7

Distributed by:
AromaTools
1-866-728-0070 / 801-798-7921
www.AromaTools.com

Table of Contents

EVERY PATIENT CARRIES
HER OR HIS OWN DOCTOR INSIDE
ALBERT SCHWEITZER

PREFACE

In her book, Knockout, Suzanne Somers discusses what she learned from interviewing doctors who are curing and preventing cancer alternatively.

When asked what the main message was that she took away from her conversations with these physicians, Suzanne responded that "the 'war on cancer' is a dismal failure. There has been no progress in curing cancer in conventional medicine for 50 years. The standard marker for success is gauged by what is called the 'surrogate end point,' which is when a tumor shrinks after four weeks, even if the patient dies in week five!"

Main revelations for Suzanne were as follows:

- There are only three types of cancers for which chemotherapy is effective.

- A popular drug has been proven ineffective in up to 92 percent of the women to whom it is given for breast cancer, yet it is still being administered.

- The conventional treatment of cancer is big business—a $200 billion a year industry—and yet conventional chemotherapy only yields a 2 percent response rate.

- There are other options.

Suzanne was diagnosed with breast cancer at age 51, so she understands how frightening and debilitating a diagnosis can be. She understands and respects patients' need to make choices for themselves regarding their personal health.

Suzanne says that "It's essential to know that cancer kills, and everyone with cancer has to recognize the seriousness of the disease and respect it." She says her book Knockout allows readers to make an informed choice to save their life. Suzanne also says that screening the documentary movie Food, Inc. made her rethink eating meat and dairy, and she recommends that everyone see it.

We have a multi-billion dollar industry that is killing people, right and left, just for financial gain. Their idea of research is to see whether two doses of this poison is better than three doses of that poison. Glen Warner, MD, Oncologist

INTRODUCTION

Most men die of their remedies, not of their illnesses. Moliere

I am a licensed massage therapist and holistic health coach and have been helping people heal ever since 1994, when I graduated from Utah College of Massage Therapy. I haven't always been interested in natural healing. In fact, until I was in my mid thirties, I was actually quite resistant to the idea that plants and other natural medicines had any real healing powers. I clumped most plant medicine and natural healing modalities into the "snake oil" category.

Eventually, my poor lifestyle habits and overuse of medicine created so many health problems that prescription and over-the-counter meds stopped helping and made me feel worse instead of better. When I first tried herbs, it was only as a last resort. A friend had been encouraging me to take herbs for months, and I only agreed because I was desperate and didn't know what else to do. I was very surprised when a week later I felt better than I'd felt in months! This totally piqued my interested in natural medicine, and graduating from massage school was only the beginning.

Over the past eighteen years, I've had the opportunity to attend a wide variety of preventive and alternative medicine trainings, which have given me a pretty good understanding of how the body works and what it needs to be healthy. And I really love it when I'm able to pass on something useful!

One of the reasons why I'm so passionate about the message in this book is because I remember how frustrated and scared I was when my doctor admitted he didn't have a solution to my health problems. I am grateful every day for the knowledge and wisdom I have gained and for "healing tools" such as herbs, essential oils, etc. that enable me to confidently and effectively manage my health at home.

Now when I get sick, which is less and less as time goes on, I'm able to dig into my healer's toolbox, so to speak, and successfully doctor myself at home. For me, home doctoring has worked so well that I haven't been to a doctor or taken prescription medicine for almost two decades, simply because I haven't needed to!

Another thing that drives me is watching really sick people suffer without even trying a natural solution simply because their belief system won't allow them to. For example, in January of 2012 on her 53rd birthday, my sister-in-law was diagnosed with stage 3 cancer. She didn't want to die and told me she was willing to try anything. I told her that frankincense essential oil has been shown in multiple scientific studies to rapidly kill cancer cells without harming healthy cells. She said she'd like to try it, so I sent her a couple of bottles along with some nutritional supplements and other essential oils known to have anticancer properties. I also sent her some books that explained the many benefits of essential oils, nutrition, and positive thinking.

When Cindy told her doctor that she was considering using essential oils, he said absolutely not. Plus, when she got the oils and smelled them, she decided they stunk. So she began several rounds of radiation and chemotherapy… as much as was allowable; and needless to say, she suffered greatly over the next couple of months. Not only was she very sick and weak, but she also lost her hair and a lot of weight. Most of the time she was in a tremendous amount of pain. Sadly, Cindy died in January of 2013, three days before her 54th birthday.

At first I was very frustrated when Cindy didn't even give frankincense a chance. I've seen miracles happen with this oil, and I truly believed it could have helped her. Then I realized that Cindy didn't share my belief system and that she was scared and doing the best she could under the circumstances. She trusted her doctor and medicine, because if she wanted to have a chance of overcoming cancer that's what her belief system said she had to do.

As I watched Cindy go through her painful ordeal, I realized that for some people the time to gain a testimony that essential oils work is not when they're critically ill and afraid.

So that, in a nutshell, explains why I'm on a mission to teach you how your body-mind-spirit works and why I'm sincerely hoping you'll open your mind to the simple truths in this book. My goal is to educate you and present you with ideas that will resonate as truth to your soul and inspire you to upgrade your habits and live a healthy and PREVENTIVE lifestyle!

I absolutely love it when someone tells me that they've taken charge of their health and turned their poor health issues around! It is so awesome to hear people's success stories! That's one of my favorite things about my work. What could be more rewarding than empowering others to be their best?

One thing I'll always be grateful for is the opportunity to help my good friend Rachel successfully rid her body of an advanced state of cancer. Rachel has been cancer-free from more than 12 years, and her experience has helped me overcome my own fears of cancer and gain a lot of confidence in the body's ability to heal even from advanced and serious diseases.

The information in this book is based on my own personal knowledge and experiences. It is not intended to diagnose, prescribe, or cure… just increase your awareness of known facts and boost your ability to take primary responsibility for your health. Plain and simple, if you are sick I hope to assist you in ridding your body of disease and creating an optimal state of being! And if you are well, my goal is to support you in staying that way.

That said, Wellness Made Simple offers a straight-up and basic approach to healing that is often pooh-poohed by health-care professionals. I've often wondered why. Perhaps its because it is too simple. Or perhaps it's because the medical profession, as a whole, is an income-generating "business," and there's no money to be made in prescribing natural and unregulated practices and substances. And healthy patients and patients who are quickly cured means business or income lost.

Now I am certainly not suggesting that doctors only care about profits. In fact, there are plenty of awesome doctors who totally have their patients' best interests at heart! What I am pointing out is that doctors are mainly trained to order tests, prescribe medicine, and perform surgeries, etc. and not to consider that there are other natural options that might actually work better for you and your budget. And there is a lot of money to be made in prescribing medicine and medical procedures.

When it comes to the medical and pharmaceutical profession, you might as well face it—it's a money-making racket. To prove this point, I have a friend who is currently dealing with breast cancer. She has chosen to deal with it by combining natural medicine with traditional medicine. In other words, she's going to a doctor and taking advice that feels right and makes sense to her, and at the same time she is using/taking therapeutic-grade essential oils and herbs as well as high quality nutritional supplements (namely frankincense, Daily Supplements, Essential Oil Cellular Complex, and Energy & Stamina Complex), which are known to increase immunity and have a positive effect on cancer cells.

Recently, I asked my friend how she was doing. Her reply was "pretty good, but it's a good thing I don't take every bit of advice a doctor gives me." She then proceeded to tell me that her regular doctor had referred her to a specialist who'd prescribed a procedure that would cost over $1,000.00 to get rid of excess estrogen. "What a rip off," my friend said as she refused the treatment and paid a hefty bill for the visit. She left the specialist's office hopping mad because in the past year several tests had shown that her body was hardly producing any estrogen at all! Later, when her regular doctor saw what the specialist has recommended, he admitted that it didn't make any sense to him either.

So, back to the subject of money making: It's a common practice for drug companies to self-fund studies that show their products are safe and beneficial, while at the same time independent researchers who are testing the very same products often get entirely different results.

Even though many studies have shown that herbs and essential oils are very safe and effective, not to mention the fact that hundreds of thousands of people have taken them with superior results and very few negative side effects, there are widely published studies which have been done by large pharmaceutical companies that have repeatedly shown herbs are "dangerous" and/or non-effective, at best.

On top of that, consumers are bombarded with misinformation by television commercials and magazine ads that continually glamorize and push "branded" and "patented" products, including medications, which are supposedly going to improve our health. Did you know that the majority of these "health-promoting" products contain cheap fillers and binders and harmful chemicals that are KNOWN to cause health problems?

I'm sure you've noticed how in ads and commercials they always show healthy-looking people enjoying life because now they are taking (whatever miracle drug) and no longer suffering from their ailment… And then, camouflaged in soft music and flowers there is a VERY LONG list of side effects that come from taking the wonder drug. How can that be good for you?

Ironically, each year Americans spend billions of dollars on branded and patented "health-related" products; yet overall, they are unhealthier than ever. I recently read that in the United States cancer has jumped from one person in eight diagnosed, to one out of three for men, and one out of two for women! These numbers are staggering! Clearly it's large corporations that are the winners here and not us, the consumers!

In spite of what commercials, advertisements, and even your doctor might be saying, the healthiest and safest substances are not patented or made in laboratories. Rather, they are God-made natural resources that have existed on the earth ever since it was created.

There is an herb or essential oil known to positively affect every condition known to man, and one single herb or oil can positively affect a wide variety of ailments, just as one ailment can be positively affected by a wide variety of herbs and essential oils! Not only do herbs and other healing plants grow easily and freely throughout the world, but they are also extremely safe, versatile, and easy to use.

At this time, herbs and nutritional supplements are unregulated; but there are groups trying to change that. Regulation wouldn't necessarily ensure better quality, it would just make it possible for the government and other vested groups to have more control—and it would drive prices up. It's much better for you and I that herbs and supplements are kept unregulated.

As a consumer, you can protect yourself by doing some homework and searching out companies that are absolutely passionate about only producing and outsourcing the highest quality herbs, essential oils, and supplements. Once you find companies you can trust, be sure to support them with your pocketbook. Your "buying power" will help keep companies who are doing it right in business!

All that said, as you read this book, please keep in mind that each body and condition is unique; therefore, the most effective form of treatment is not going to be the same for everyone. No one knows what your body needs to heal better than you do, except God, who created you and knows everything about you. So when seeking healing, it's best to research all of your options and then prayerfully choose the best approach to take… and then follow your gut (especially after praying), because your gut will almost always steer you right.

Most diseases are the result of medication which has been prescribed to relieve and take away a beneficent and warning symptom on the part of Nature. Elbert Hubbard

DISEASE AND HEALING MADE SIMPLE

So many [doctors] come to the sickroom thinking of themselves as men of science fighting disease and not as healers with a little knowledge helping nature to get a sick man well.
Sir Auckland Geddes

Disease, or a state of "dis-ease" in the body, is not a random thing. It is a result of cause and effect. Likewise, healing does not come from covering up or "Band-Aiding" symptoms. Taking a "pill to fit the ill" will never really cure disease. In order to heal disease at its roots where it started, you must backtrack and clean up what created it in the first place.

Wellness Made Simple addresses cancer specifically because cancer is a low-level, bottom-of-the-disease-chain, condition, and taking steps to prevent or cure cancer will help you prevent and cure other diseases as well.

Healing is fairly easy once you understand the basics:

• "Disease" simply indicates a state of physical, emotional, and/or spiritual distress—something's not at ease… It's in a state of dis-ease.

• Pain is a signal that something is wrong or out of balance.

• Fevers, colds, flu, and any type of oozing or draining condition, including throwing up and bleeding without a cut, are the body's way of cleansing a toxic and overloaded system.

• Medicines might make symptoms go away, but they can't solve problems at their roots where they originated. In fact, medicine is toxic and causes side effects and further imbalance and usually leads to more health problems down the road. Taking a pill can't fix the illness because medicine cannot cure disease!

• The only way to truly heal disease is to address it at its roots... and clean up what created it in the first place.

Healing is fairly easy once you understand that problematic conditions occur when the body-mind-spirit becomes imbalanced and stays that way for an extended period of time. The main trick for healing and maintaining good health is simply to create and maintain balance. When the body is in balance, it is in what's referred to as "homeostasis," which is what enables the body to self-heal.

So, how do you create homeostasis? You upgrade your habits! Seriously, diseases like cancer, heart disease, and diabetes can be largely predicted just by observing a person's dietary and other living habits. Many studies have shown that people who eat right and exercise and drink enough water and get enough sleep and have positive, happy attitudes rarely have health problems. Whereas people with sluggish routines and poor eating, exercise, and sleep habits and negative and depressed attitudes often get sick—and they are also prone to develop serious illnesses!

Adopting a healthy lifestyle is your main tool for preventing and curing disease. When it comes to taking care of your body, an ounce of prevention is worth much more than a pound of cure! It's super important to take good care of yourself in the first place, because once a problem becomes set, it's much harder to heal it.

So how can you tell if something's out of whack? If your body is in pain or oozing or burning up or lethargic or icy cold or if you're more than a little bit overweight or have sores or rashes that won't heal or you feel exhausted and depressed and constantly have a headache, it is not normal! Your body-mind-spirit is trying to tell you that something is wrong, and it needs you to pay attention and give it what it needs so it can become balanced.

I don't suggest waiting for your doctor to confirm that something is wrong, and here's why: A condition has to be about 60 percent along in the body before it can even be detected by a blood test. Based on that, if you're body is trying to tell you there is a problem, by the time your doctor tells you that something is wrong, it just might be too late. The sooner you can get on something and turn it around, the better!

The time to take control of your health and adopt a wellness lifestyle is now, before you get sick. If your body is sending you signals that something is wrong, don't wait. Get on it now, and do whatever you can (today) to take care of the issue and reverse it while it's still in the beginning stages. If you are already very sick and have been given little hope, don't give up! Remember the body-mind-spirit has an amazing ability to restore itself and heal and that miracles happen all the time. Have faith (prayer is very helpful), and do whatever you can to support your entire system in restoring itself to health.

If you have been diagnosed with a label disease, such as cancer, type 2 diabetes, ADD/ADHD, fibromyalgia, Parkinson's, multiple sclerosis, or an autoimmune disease such as lupus, your body is screaming at you that it is toxic and seriously out of balance! And it needs you to help it get to homeostasis... so it can start to self-heal!

The good news is that the human body-mind-spirit is so resilient and repairable that with some help—take the bad stuff out and put a lot of good stuff in—most people's bodies and brains will quickly respond and begin to self-heal.

If you want to become healthier, you must do things that create and restore harmony and balance within your body-mind-spirit, including releasing destructive generational (energetic) patterns and fearful, hopeless, negative emotions. And, just so you know, this requires spiritual assistance; therefore I recommend that you sincerely pray for help!

If you are reading this and feeling overwhelmed because the thought of overhauling your lifestyle seems daunting and unappealing, I just want you to know that I can totally relate! In fact, I'd probably still be doing things the same old way, except doing what I was doing was creating a host of health problem. And I didn't like the way I felt. And I wasn't willing to resign myself to a variety of "label diseases" and a life of doctors, pills, and increased sickness (not to mention out of control medical bills). So I chose to look for new and healthier ways to care for myself. And the good news is that the natural ways have worked so well that I haven't looked back. And, I have found that instead of being hard and overwhelming (like I originally thought), taking good care of myself is actually a whole lot easier and more rewarding than always feeling tired and sick was!

So, here's what my experiences have taught me: We are not merely victims to our circumstances; but rather, God our creator has endowed us with self-healing bodies and minds as well as limitless potential and resources so that we can rise up and overcome poor health and circumstances! I strongly believe that most of what we experience is the result of cause and effect. In other words, there are consequences. And if we don't like what we're getting, all we have to do is make different choices so that we will get different results.

Some people are more than ready to take charge of their health. They are totally open to holistic medicine and welcome new ideas and information. Other people are skeptical and unwilling to unplug from the brainwashed belief that they need a (money-making) system to heal them. They have little or no faith in their body's ability to self-heal and don't believe that living a more natural (earthy and spiritual) lifestyle will help them. No matter where you stand, I invite you to keep reading with an open mind. I hope something in this book will ring true and inspire you to live a healthier, happier, and more rewarding life!

Medicine being a compendium of the successive and contradictory mistakes of medical practitioners, when we summon the wisest of them to our aid, the chances are that we may be relying on a scientific truth the error of which will be recognized in a few years' time. Marcel Proust

CANCER IN A NUTSHELL

The concept of total wellness recognizes that our every thought, word, and behavior affects our greater health and well-being. And we, in turn, are affected not only emotionally but also physically and spiritually. Greg Anderson

Sometimes our time is up and dying from cancer is the will of God, and there is nothing that can be done to prevent it. But, most of the time this is not the case, and it is well within our realm to heal—especially when cancer is still in the beginning stages.

As far as healing goes, it's important that you understand that when the human body is in a balanced state, it has the ability to keep itself healthy and quickly heal itself. It is also important to realize that as far as medicine goes, medicine, in and of itself, does not have the ability to heal the body. Medicine can be very useful for temporarily taking away pain and also for stabilizing traumatized bodies and saving lives. But medicine cannot cure cancer or any other form of disease, and, overall, it weakens the body and creates further states of disharmony and distress. The fact that many people actually recover after receiving harsh chemical treatments such as chemotherapy and radiation is a testimony to the body's amazing ability to heal and restore itself.

When dealing with cancer and other diseases, it's important to address the problem early on and then use the wonderful plants and other natural resources that God has given us to restore our bodies to a harmonious and healthy balanced state—so they can begin the internal process of self-healing.

Cancer can start anywhere in the body. It is defined as a malignant growth or tumor caused by abnormal and uncontrolled cell division. There are approximately 200 known types of cancer, and certain types of body tissue are prone to attract specific cancers more than other types are. For instance, smoking is known to cause lung and throat cancer, while nitrates are strongly linked to pancreatic cancer. And soy, birth-control pills, and hormone replacement therapy (increased estrogen) are strongly linked to breast and uterine cancers.

The main difference between normal cells and cancerous cells is this: In cancerous cells, some of the genes have been damaged. This causes the cells to send out incorrect signals, which, in turn, causes cells to divide improperly. Normal cells double 50 or 60 times and then they die; but cancer cells don't follow this pattern. Instead, they continue to double and multiply and spread rapidly. Cancer cells typically self-destruct more slowly than they reproduce. And so their numbers continue to increase or "mutate" until eventually there are billions of copies of the original cancerous cell. These clusters of cancerous cells then form into cancerous tumors.

Cancer starts with changes in one cell or a small group of cells. Typically, cancerous cells have been reproducing out of control long before a lump can be detected by a doctor or seen on a scan. Once cancer or mutated cells become set in the body, they can rapidly spread to other parts of the body through the lymphatic system.

However, in the beginning it's not easy for mutated cells to take hold. When mutated cells first form, the immune system often recognizes them as abnormal cells and destroys them. Cells often self-destruct when they're carrying a mutation. This means that most precancerous cells die before they can turn into cancer. As bodies break down with age or become weakened through unhealthy lifestyles, it's easier for mutations to occur and for cancer cells to develop. This is why older people and people who haven't practiced healthy lifestyles have an increased risk of getting cancer.

CANCER CELLS SIMPLIFIED

Time is amazingly forgiving. No matter how much time you've wasted in the past, you still have an entire today.
Dennis Waitley

A "cell nucleus" has the job of controlling gene expression. Genes are coded messages inside cells that tell the cells what to do. There are three types of genes involved in cancer: tumor suppressor genes, DNA repair genes, and oncogenes.

•TUMOR SUPPRESSOR GENES stop cells from multiplying needlessly. When tumor suppressor genes become damaged and stop working, cells are able to continually multiply without dying like they are supposed to die.

•DNA REPAIR GENES normally repair damage done to the DNA; but when these genes become damaged, a cell may not repair mutations—instead, it is able to copy the mutations into new cells.

•ONCOGENES are abnormal genes that encourage cells to multiply. The cells in healthy adults don't multiply much except to repair damage, such as healing a cut or wound. But when genes become abnormal, they tell the cell to multiply and divide all the time.

Normal cells stick together in the right place and reproduce themselves exactly. They become specialized or mature, and then they stop reproducing at the right time. They self-destruct and die if they are damaged.

Cancer cells do not stick together and stay where they're supposed to. This enables them to quickly travel to other parts of the body. They don't participate in the "signaling system" of normal cells either; rather, they tend to send the signal to other cells to continue to fire and reproduce. Cancer cells also become less mature as they age. This is because they reproduce so often that their genetic information is lost. Cancer cells reproduce even more rapidly and haphazardly with time.

When cells are looked at through a microscope, cancer cells can be distinguished from normal cells. If cancer cells are similar looking to normal cells, it is determined that the cancer is at a low or "level 1" stage.

If cancer cells are large and irregular, it means they are "advanced"—and the cancer is referred to as "stage 3" or "stage 4." Usually, the further advanced cancer cells are, the more rapidly they spread throughout the body.

Finding a cure for cancer is absolutely contraindicated by the profits of the cancer industry's chemotherapy, radiation, and surgery cash trough. Dr. Diamond, MD, and Ross Horne, Health and Survival in the 21st Century

CREATING WELLNESS

I cannot tell you that if you do everything I've suggested in this book it will cure you of cancer. What I can say is that it is possible to support the human body in self-healing from even serious conditions like cancer without involving toxic drugs, vaccines, or surgery.

When it comes to the human body, there are three main things to remember:

1. An unbalanced body is weak and susceptible to disease.

2. A balanced body is strong and healthy.

3. The human body is extremely resilient and repairable.

So, if you have an unbalanced and unhealthy body and want to turn it around, you need to get the bad stuff out and put a lot of good stuff in. If you do this, it's very likely your body will respond and begin to heal. The good news is that there are numerous inexpensive and effective things you can do to get bad stuff out and put good stuff in, or in other words to restore homeostasis or balance.

Now here's what you need to remember about cancer: Cancer is synonymous with Candida yeast, low oxygen, low frequencies (energy), and high acidity. Cancer thrives in an acidic and yeasty body, but it cannot grow in an alkaline and oxygenated system. In order for mutated cells to take hold in the body, the body has to be quite acidic and weak. Therefore, it makes sense that a first step would be to take aggressive steps to restore alkalinity and, in addition, do whatever it takes to raise your frequency and oxygenate your cells.

If you have any type of cancer, it's a given that you have a prolific overgrowth of Candida yeast, your energy is low, and your cells are deprived of oxygen.

In a nutshell, here's what's important to do:

1. Alkalize your system.

2. Oxygenate your system.

3. Raise your body's frequency.

Keep reading, and I'll teach you how...

THINGS THAT ARE KNOWN TO CAUSE CANCER

There are certain activities, substances, and behaviors that are known to create weakness and imbalance in the body and to cause it to break down to the point that cells begin to malfunction and divide improperly. If you look at this list, you'll see that it's unwholesome, unnatural, and unproductive things, whether they be physical or mental, that are known to cause cancer.

• Negative and angry outlook on life (victim mentality); harboring toxic emotions such as jealously, resentment, and guilt
• Alcohol consumption
• Anxiety and stress; an overly stressed or impaired immune system
• Artificial hormone therapy, including birth control pills
• Candida yeast—a lethargic and acidic system
• Carcinogens (exposure to things known to cause cancer)
• Chlorine
• Chronic stress
• Diets high in saturated and trans fats (dairy, meat, junk food)
• Excessive tanning and overexposure to the sun
• Exposure to chemicals (including preservatives, pesticides, and chemicals found in household cleaners and hygiene products)
• Exposure to low frequencies (low energy)
• Fluoride
• Genetic makeup (like you are born with a loaded gun…. Still, you must pull the trigger with a poor lifestyle for the gun to go off)
• Lethargy (feeling lifeless/super low oxygen state)
• Low oxygen in the cells
• Microwaved food (especially when eaten on a regular basis)
• Obesity (EXCESS baggage weighing you down)

- Overly concerned with others needs—lack of self-nurturing
- Poor diet (processed, fake, clogging, and dead foods)
- Smoking and cigarette smoke
- Sodium nitrate (harmful preservatives)
- Sugar! (Cancer absolutely thrives on it—sugar is cancer food)
- Toxic environment (mental and physical)
- Weakened immunity

*The thousand mysteries around us would not trouble but in-
terest us, if only we had cheerful, healthy hearts.*
Friedrich Wilhelm Nietzsche

WHAT'S KNOWN TO PREVENT AND HEAL CANCER

- A happy, positive, grateful (non-toxic) attitude
- Cleansing—ridding the body of toxins (create alkalinity)
- Therapeutic-grade essential oils (They oxygenate & support cells)
- Eating mainly a raw food, plant-based diet, combined with high quality nutritional supplements
- Enthusiasm—love and appreciation for life!
- Forgiveness (letting things go and choosing love)
- Herbs (They cleanse and balance the body)
- Healthy fats
- Heartfelt prayer
- Juicing/drinking lots of green smoothies
- Laughter
- Light
- Living a wellness or preventative lifestyle
- Love
- Meditation and guided imagery
- Oxygenating cells
- Regular cardiovascular exercise
- Keeping frequencies high
- Taking/eating herbs and spices

Health is a state of complete physical, mental, and social well-being and not merely the absence of disease or infirmity.
World Health Organization, 1948

BREAKING DOWN THE CAUSES

Sickness is poor-spirited, and cannot serve anyone; it must husband its resources to live. But health or fullness answers its own ends, and has to spare, runs over, and inundates the neighborhoods and creeks of other men's necessities.
Ralph Waldo Emerson

● CANDIDA YEAST—AN ACIDIC SYSTEM!
A growing body of scientific evidence shows that there is an overgrowth of Candida yeast (and resulting acidity) behind all forms of cancer. So it doesn't make much sense that chemotherapy and radiation, which actually feed Candia yeast, are the most common form of medical treatment. In 1993, it was stated in Contemporary Oncology Magazine (USA) that "Cancer patients undergoing radio or chemotherapy did not finally succumb to the cancer itself, but to an infestation of Candida albicans."

Candida (Candida albicans) is one of the many types of microorganisms/parasites that naturally live in the digestive tract. In a healthy digestive tract, there is a ratio of one yeast cell (harmful bacteria) per one million probiotic cells (beneficial bacteria). Under this properly-balanced condition, Candida has to fight to survive. However, when the bacteria balance in the digestive tract becomes imbalanced, or the intestinal pH becomes too acidic, it creates a perfect environment for yeast to grow and thrive and candidiasis results—and immune system functioning is impaired. In other words, candidiasis, or overgrown yeast, is a state of having more harmful bacteria than beneficial bacteria in the digestive tract.

The digestive tract is lined with a protective mucus membrane that is damaged by candidiasis. When yeast becomes prolific, it changes from a yeast form to a fungal form that grows roots that excrete acid. The acidic roots puncture the mucus lining, which enables bacteria, yeast, toxins, undigested food particles, and fecal matter to pass through into the bloodstream. This condition, which is often referred to as leaky gut syndrome, is harmful to the body and can make a person very ill.

More serious, once fungal forms of Candidia yeast are released into the blood stream, they begin to attack the cells and damage them and cause them to divide improperly and send incorrect signals.

Chemotherapy and radiation are the most common forms of medical treatment for cancer, and yet they feed Candida yeast, which feeds cancer. It's no wonder in 1993 that Contemporary Oncology Magazine (USA) stated, "Cancer patients undergoing radio or chemotherapy did not finally succumb to the cancer itself, but to an infestation of Candida albicans." Prescription medicine can't cure candidiasis or the diseases it causes, but instead they add fuel to the fire and make unfavorable conditions much worse.

If you have cancer, one of the most inexpensive and effective things you can do is go on (and stay on) a yeast-free diet!

● BIRTH CONTROL PILLS AND ARTIFICIAL HORMONES
In 2003, for the first time in over a decade, breast cancer was shown to be on a decline. This was significant because it followed the news that "hormone treatments cause an increase in breast cancer." After the announcement, sales of Prempo, the prescribed hormone therapy drug for menopausal women, dropped in half.

Artificial hormones of all types should be avoided, including the hormones that are liberally pumped into meat and dairy products. Almost all meat and dairy is loaded with artificial hormones, which are strongly linked to cancer and other health problems. Even products labeled as hormone- and antibiotic-free can still contain up to ten percent.

• STRESS

Prolonged feelings of stress and anxiety create chaos in the body and lead to health problems, including adrenal burn-out, allergies, depression, fatigue, ulcers, and heart disease. Perpetual states of stress lead to hormone imbalances (in-creased estrogen and decreased progesterone stores) and digestive problems—which all feed Candida yeast and can eventually lead to cancer. The next time you feel yourself get-ting uptight, try releasing tension by listening to funny stories and/or uplifting music and/or singing, breathing, exercising, drawing, coloring, or writing your anxiety out.

• JUNK FOODS AND PROCESSED FAKE FOODS (SOFT DRINKS, COFFEE, ETC.)

Professor Will Steward, a top professor of oncology at Leices-ter Royal Infirmary, has warned that junk food and fizzy drink diets may be leading to the rise in bowel cancer among younger people. Dr. Steward spoke out after studies revealed that the number of people under 30 with bowel cancer has doubled in the past decade. He encouraged young people to cut out fast food and soft/energy drinks, saying, "These fig-ures are extremely worrying. People under 30 don't expect to get colon cancer. It is far more common in people over 70 and is thought of as an old people's cancer." If you are concerned about cancer and other diseases, it is imperative that you wean yourself and your family off of fake food, including fast foods, processed foods, candy, energy drinks, sports drinks, soft drinks, coffee and sugary coffee drinks, etc.

• SMOKING AND SECOND-HAND CIGARETTE SMOKE

It's common knowledge that smoking greatly increases the risk of lung cancer, but did you know that studies have shown that non-smokers who inhale cigarette smoke on a regular basis have a 25 percent greater chance of getting lung cancer than people who don't breathe in second-hand smoke?

● ALCOHOL
A study of 1.2 million middle-aged women done in the UK shows that drinking alcoholic beverages increases women's risk of getting cancer. In the study, women who only had one alcoholic drink a day (beer, wine, or hard liquor) were still found to be at an increased risk of getting cancers of the liver, rectum, breast, mouth, and esophagus.

● DIETS HIGH IN SUGAR AND SATURATED/TRANS FATS
The same major European study mentioned above showed that women with raised blood sugar levels have a significantly greater risk of developing cancers of the pancreas, skin, womb, and urinary tract. And women who eat high levels of unhealthy fats (38 percent of their daily diets) have an increased risk of developing breast cancer. In addition, a U.S. study also found that older women with fatty diets (40 percent of their daily diets) have an increased chance of developing breast cancer (Google "Million women study in the UK").

● OBESITY
Research done at the University of California in San Diego confirmed that obesity acts as a "bona fide tumor promoter" (Cell, January 22, 2010). In this study, researchers discovered that liver cancer is fostered by inflammation in the body—which goes hand in hand with obesity and imbalanced and critically hot and inflamed organs. If you have too much body fat, losing weight and cleansing can help you reduce your risk of getting cancer and other debilitating diseases. Drinking green drinks (smoothies) will help you shed fat and cleanse toxins.

• MICROWAVES

Microwaves are convenient and fast, but microwave cooking isn't nearly as good as it seems. Here's a short explanation of how microwaves work and why they are so bad for you. Microwave ovens contain magnetrons, or tubes in which electrons are affected by magnetic and electric fields in such a way that they produce microwave-length radiation. This microwave energy changes polarity from positive to negative millions of times every second. Because microwaves are generated from the magnetron, the electromagnetic rays bombard whatever's in the oven (food and water) and cause its molecules to rotate at their same frequency. This agitation creates molecular friction that heats up food quickly, but it also tears food molecules apart and damages them.

In the book The True Messages in Water, Masaru Emoto uses pictures to illustrate how microwaves destroy the integrity of water. After water is microwaved, it takes on a round shape and will no longer form into crystals. Microwaves create unknown byproducts in food that the body cannot metabolize or break down. They are known to demagnetize brain tissue and cause immune system deficiencies, cancerous cells in human blood, and cancerous growths in the stomach and intestine. The ill effects of microwaved food byproducts are residual (long-term and permanent) within the human body. Williams Sonoma stores do not sell microwaves. This is because the company's founders have chosen not to market them because they believe microwaves "not only affect the taste of the food, but also present 'safety concerns' for the food itself."

• CHLORINE

Since the beginning of the 19th century, chlorine bleach has been routinely added to U.S. drinking water simply because it's the cheapest means of disinfection. According to the U.S.

Council of Environmental Quality, "Cancer risk among people drinking chlorinated water is 93 percent higher than among those whose water does not contain chlorine." If you are buying bottled water, you should know that distilled water is a safer and healthier choice than most bottled water, which typically contains pollutants. If you are concerned about chlorine absorbtion from bathwater, you can prevent it by installing a filter on your showerhead.

● EXPOSURE TO CHEMICALS
Fluorinated polymers are commonly used in things like microwave popcorn bags, fast-food wrappers, stain-free carpets, and windshield washer fluid. Fluorinated polymers degrade to become a group of toxic chemicals called perfluorocarboxylates (PFCAs), which are linked to cancer and other development disorders. What's most alarming about PFCA's is that toxic effects are shown to be very widespread and long lasting, and high concentrations are showing up worldwide in soil and dust, as well as in the blood of animals and humans.

Fluorinated polymers are only one of a long list of toxic chemicals that are commonly found in household cleaners and hygiene and beauty products. Hygiene and beauty products typically contain a slew of toxic chemicals and hormone disrupters that are linked to many types of cancers. For this reason, it is recommended that you research companies and support only those who are passionate about producing chemical-free products. Or, make your own safe cleaners and beauty products at home. (My book, Super Simple Wellness, contains many recipes as well as in-depth information about harmful chemicals)

● SODIUM NITRATE
Sodium nitrate is a preservative that turns colorless old meat bright red and makes it more appealing. Even though

it's known to be toxic and highly carcinogenic, it is found in almost all processed meats and meats sold in stores. The USDA tried to ban sodium nitrate in the 70s but was vetoed by food manufacturers who complained that they had no alternatives for packaged meat products. Sodium nitrate adversely affects the liver and pancreas and is strongly linked to pancreatic and liver cancer.

- SOY AND SOY PRODUCTS
Soy has long been touted as a healthy meat and dairy alternative that helps prevent breast cancer, but in reality, soy beans and soy products are far from healthy. In fact, a lot of independent research done on soy has shown that it is one of the highest foods in phytoestrogens, which are plant-based estrogens that mimic estrogen in our bodies.

Estrogen dominance is a leading cause of breast cancer, endometriosis, uterine fibroids, infertility, and low libido. It is caused by foods high in estrogen, including soy. Soy consumption also has an extremely adverse effect on children. For instance, when an infant drinks the daily-recommended amount of soy formula, he or she consumes a hormone load equivalent to four birth control pills! Soy consumption has been connected to autoimmune and thyroid problems in infants, stunted growth in babies and children, a shockingly large number of girls starting their periods at age 6 and 7, and the high infertility rate among young couples desiring to get pregnant.

- AN IMPAIRED IMMUNE SYSTEM
Live blood analysis enable us to clearly see the differences between healthy and impaired immune systems. In a strong and healthy immune system, the white blood cells are separate and round with a ring of light around them (oxygenated), and they're freely moving around. But in an underactive and

suppressed immune system, the white blood cells are close together and stacked up sideways and on top of each other in tight rows (like Pringles), and they are lying very still, as if they're trying to protect themselves.

Blood cells need oxygen to thrive; and in order for cells to receive oxygen, they must have space around them. When blood cells are stacked up tight in neat little rows, they don't have much surface space, and they can't absorb much oxygen.

• LOW OXYGEN IN CELLS
Normal cells need oxygen to function properly, but cancer cells actually thrive when they are oxygen deficient. Blood needs oxygen to the extent that when the capillary system is deprived of oxygen it can easily become cancerous. In fact, when the level of saturation falls below about 60 percent, it creates an optimal environment for cells to go haywire and mutate. Getting regular aerobic exercise is one of the best ways to oxygenate your blood. Drinking raw green drinks like wheatgrass juice or green smoothies, breathing deeply, and drinking oxygenated water (like Kangen water) also helps oxygenate blood.

• LACK OF EXERCISE
In 2001, a panel of international experts from the World Health Organization evaluated a lack of exercise in relation to cancer. Their research showed that exercising to keep weight within a healthy range reduces the risk of getting certain types of cancer, specifically breast and colon cancer, and possibly endometrial and prostate cancer.

• LOW FREQUENCIES
There is a growing body of evidence that shows a strong correlation between high frequencies and good health and low fre-

quencies and disease. The higher the frequency, the healthier and happier we are; but the lower the frequency, the worse we feel and the faster our cells and tissues deteriorate and break down. Constant exposure to things such as negative people and thoughts, junk food, degrading music and movies, and excessively loud and irritating noise depletes us and makes us more susceptible to cancer and other types of disease.

• IRRESPONSIBLE SEX
Having unprotected sex has been shown to cause sexually transmitted diseases and an increased risk of adnormal cell growth and cervical cancer. The risk is especially high among young people, people who have had sex with multiple partners, and women who have sex with men who have had multiple partners.

• EXTREME TANNING AND SUN EXPOSURE
Tanning is the process of browning the skin by exposure to the sun or ultraviolet lights. Each year, approximately 30 million Americans visit tanning salons. This averages out to about be about 1 million tanning salons visits per day. A 20-minute session in a tanning bed is equivalent to 4 hours of unprotected sun outside. While getting too much sun (or spending too much time in a tanning bed) on a regular basis, and repeatedly getting sunburned, can cause skin cancer, it's been shown that moderate unprotected exposure to sunlight or UVA and UVB rays can actually help prevent cancer (this is not well-known, but true). Thus occasional tanning sessions are not a bad thing. But overdoing it can cause problems—especially if you have an overloaded and weakened immune system.

• AN ANGRY AND NEGATIVE OUTLOOK ON LIFE
Your emotions have a tremendous impact on your health.

Here's why: feeling angry and bitter and carrying a chip on your shoulder is not a happy, healthy, or normal state. The main problem with having an angry countenance and/or victim mentality (besides the fact that it makes you feel miserable and look unattractive) is that it impairs your immune function and inhibits the natural release of healthy feel-good hormones. This creates a lethargic and stagnant environment that's perfect for Candida yeast and mutating cells.

EXAMINING WHAT HEALS

The secret is in getting your body so chemically "unloaded" and "nutrient primed" that it heals itself. The challenge is that all chemicals are inorganic in nature, and the body, by itself, can only metabolize material that is organic. We need help, and nature itself has provided an answer. Nature has within it some phenomenal, organic nutrients that have high chemical detoxifying properties that are also very powerful mineralizers, oxygenators, antioxidants and immune boosters, as well as, very powerful bioavailable nutrition. Sherry A, Rogers MD

- CLEANSING
Constipation, bloating, excessive gassiness, and Candida yeast are all symptoms of a dirty colon. Though not so obvious, depression, headaches, fatigue, anxiety, poor circulation, back pain, high-blood pressure, low libido, obesity, poor concentration, allergies, and swollen legs are also conditions caused by a gunky digestive system. A clean digestive tract is vitally important to good health because toxicity in the digestive tract is linked to pretty much all disease, including colon cancer, which is second only to lung cancer among cancer deaths in the United States!

Cleansing removes accumulated wastes from the body and frees organs from their routine chores of digestion so they can focus on really cleaning house. Cleansing enables the body to regain vitality and health. If you are very toxic, it's good to start out with the yeast-free diet combined with a gentle herbal or essential oil cleanse. Adding approximately 5–12 drops of lemon essential oil to pure water (distilled of alkalized) daily is highly recommended. This will balance your pH and gently cleanse your liver.

● A PLANT-BASED, RAW FOOD DIET
Eating a mainly raw whole food diet, including an abundance of organic dark green lettuce, spinach, kale, Swiss chard, and other color-intense fruits and vegetables, will go a long ways towards healing your body and restoring vibrant health. In addition to being loaded with vitamins and minerals, raw fruits and vegetables contain enzymes and antioxidants which protect the body against cancer and other diseases and are essential for digestion and almost all body functions. Plus, raw veggies create alkalinity—which is an optimal cancer-fighting condition in the body.

● JUICING AND GREEN SMOOTHIES
Drinking fresh juice and green smoothies is one of best things you can do for your health. Raw juice will fill you up and satisfy your body's nutritional needs, and it will help reduce your cravings for junk food. It will also make you feel and look your vibrant best. Drinking fresh juice is so good for you that you will immediately notice the benefits. Fresh, homemade juices are a far cry from store-bought bottled juices which bear little resemblance to the healthy-looking fruits and vegetables on their labels—and the same goes for smoothies loaded with sugar and artificial flavorings. Even though high-quality juicers and blenders are pricy, if you consider all the money you'll

save on visits to the doctor, medicine, and beauty treatments to make you look firmer and younger, you'll see that they are a wise investment that pays off nicely in the end!

• HERBS AND SPICES
Herbs and spices have more disease-fighting antioxidants than do most fruits and vegetables. They are very versatile, easy to use, and relatively inexpensive, which makes them ideal for fighting disease and improving health. Multiple studies have shown that herbs have unprecedented medicinal properties. Not only is each individual herb a rich source of vitamins and minerals, but, collectively, herbs have the ability to heal every disease known to man—and to fix the problems that man-made medicines create. Research done at Georgetown University shows that herbs and spices are powerful antibiotics, blood thinners, anticancer agents, anti-inflammatory agents, insulin regulators, and antioxidants, even when they're only consumed in small amounts!

• GOOD FATS INCLUDING CoQ10 AND OMEGA 3
Unlike bad fats, which clog our arteries and increase our risk of diabetes, cancer, and heart disease, good fats play an important part in a healthy diet because they are a great source of energizing fuel. Good fats transport protein and vitamins essential for nutrient absorption into the cells. Good fats assist with nerve transmission and maintaining cell membrane integrity, and they lubricate our joints and keep our skin soft, supple, and glowing.

• OXYGENATED CELLS
People with various degenerative diseases are often found to have low venous oxygen saturation. Increasing oxygen to the cells causes venous oxygen saturation levels to rise and causes health and vitality to improve dramatically. Liquid oxygen and ox-

ygen therapies work well for people who are ill, but if you are in relatively good shape and eating plenty of raw dark-green leafy veggies, doing aerobic exercise regularly, and practicing deep breathing, those things will keep your cells oxygenated.

● REGULAR EXERCISE
Physical movement is an essential part of a healthy lifestyle. Your body was designed to move! Thus, taking time to exercise should be a part of your day. Regular movement boosts sluggish immune systems and fixes unhealthy conditions such as circulation problems and weak and atrophied muscles.

● MEDITATION AND GUIDED IMAGERY
The mind is a very powerful and effective tool for healing. By simply quieting your mind for a period of time, or by using guided imagery and visualization to achieve a desired outcome, it is possible to successfully release unproductive programming (like fear) and facilitate healing miracles.

● HIGH FREQUENCIES
High-frequency substances and activities enliven us. They lift us energetically (raise our frequencies) and positively affect our health. Simple things like using pure therapeutic grade essential oils and high-quality herbs and homeopathic remedies, eating "vibrant foods" (such as fresh organic fruits and vegetables), listening to classical and upbeat music, exercising (dancing, skating, skiing, yoga, etc.), performing heartfelt acts of service, wholeheartedly participating in prayer and other spiritual practices (including reading scriptures and meditating), being honest, kind, forgiving (of self and others), and loving at heart, and having hope, faith, and charity. . . all uplift us and energize us at all levels—and consequently make us much happier and healthier than we would be otherwise!

- HEARTFELT PRAYER

The act of sincere and heartfelt prayer, whether for ourselves (petitionary prayers) or for others (intercessory prayers), has positive and healing effects. Prayer helps us feel less lonely, less agitated, and less dissatisfied. It boosts our morale and enhances our ability to cope. It lowers our blood pressure and strengthens our immune systems and helps us heal more quickly from things like alcoholism, drug addiction, surgery, and depression. Studies show that prayer is a healing balm that opens doors and connects all the pieces and makes everything come together and work more efficiently on our behalf.

- LOVE!

Love is a powerful emotion that relieves pain and increases health. People who LOVE are happier and healthier because love goes both ways. When you really love others, they tend to automatically love you back, and you reap the rewards of less stress, more joy, more contentment, more purpose, and better health, etc.

- LIGHT

Exposure to LIGHT is a powerful from of treatment for cancer. Cancer cells have been shown to immediately begin to self-destruct when they're exposed to bright light! Bright light in the form of strong sunlight, light tables, light wands, and even occasional trips to a tanning bed has been shown to be an effective aid in treating cancer.

- LAUGHTER

Laughter may very possibly be the ultimate medicine because it's absolutely free, and it's so simple that anyone and everyone can do it! Laughter has a powerful healing effect on the mind and body. Did you see The Secret? Remember the woman who cured herself of cancer just by watching comedies every night (laughing!) and repeatedly telling herself that she was in great health!

● A HAPPY AND POSITIVE ATTITUDE
People who choose to be outgoing and positive are typically happy and content with their circumstances, regardless of what they are. But negative and discontent people tend to complain and be unhappy, no matter how good their circumstances are.

The main difference between happy and unhappy people is that happy people see the bright side of things and bloom, rather than wilt, where they're planted. And their ability to be optimistic and adaptable, no matter what, nets them better health (less stress) and more rewarding experiences and relationships—as well as an increase in things to be happy about!

● ZERO-POINT ENERGY
In physics, zero-point energy is the lowest measurement of energy possible. It is the amount of energy associated with a vacuum of empty space. What's amazing and very cool about zero-point energy is that it can be harnessed into devices that turn on the body's own internal source energy, and, thus, it can be used to increase cellular health, reverse aging, and heal disease!

NON-NUTRITIOUS & HARMFUL FOODS

• PROCESSED CONVENIENCE FOODS

Convenience or processed foods can be eaten right out of the package or popped in the microwave and heated up in no time without dirtying a dish. Convenience foods are no-hassle time savers, for sure. What's not so great about them is that they're dead, non-nutritive foods laced with harmful chemicals. And they are proven to destroy good health and to cause obesity.

Food manufacturers routinely add additives, artificial flavorings, sweeteners, and preservatives to improve the taste of d and extend its shelf life. Many people are sensitive to food ditives but don't connect feeling bad to what they're eating. If od doesn't rot on the shelf, it won't rot in your stomach either, hich can cause a ton of health problems. MSG, artificial and atural flavors, sodium dioxide, sodium benzoate, and sodium itrate are common additives that should always be avoided. Get in the habit of reading labels before you put foods and beverages in your cart. Stay away from things that contain ng lists of nonfood ingredients you can't pronounce, including natural flavorings." Keep in mind that the shorter and simpler the label, the better. It's best to make it a practice to avoid processed and packaged foods altogether!

• SODAS (SOFT DRINKS)

Soft drinks contain water, carbon dioxide, artificial flavors, colors, acidulants, preservatives, potassium, sodium, regular or low-calorie sweeteners, and often caffeine. All ingredients are approved by the FDA. The soft-drink industry would have you believe sodas are harmless and even joy enhancing, but the truth is soft drinks are highly addictive and extremely harmful to the body. Just one soft drink contains enough sugar to immobilize the immune system by about 33 percent. And studies have shown that drinking just one soft drink a day increases children's chance of becoming obese by 60 percent! Diet soft drinks are even worse than regular sodas because they contain lab-produced sweeteners that are known to be far more harmful than normal white sugar! When it comes to soft drinks, they're all bad news!

● CAFFINATED DRINKS—ENERGY DRINKS
Caffeine is advertised as an alertness booster and a health- and athletic-performance enhancer, but while it can temporarily yield increased alertness and energy, it is definitely not a health aid. In truth, caffeine is a very addictive central nervous system stimulant that produces unnatural highs and then, when a person is coming down and off of it, headaches, sluggishness, light-headedness, depression, fatigue, and strong cravings for more.

Caffeine greatly impairs the nervous and immune systems. Excessive caffeine use is linked to low metabolism, sleep deprivation, osteoporosis, elevated blood pressure, gastrointestinal disorders, ADD/ADHD, and depression. High doses can cause potentially serious side effects such as increased heart rate, muscle twitching, jitteriness, anxiety, irritability, nervousness, acid reflux, insomnia, hypertension, and severe dehydration.

● ALCOHOL
Alcohol is an addictive drug. Alcohol consumption is attributed to about $15 billion in health care costs annually. In the short run, physical problems include reduced physical coordination, reduced mental alertness, poor decision making, staggering, slurred speech, double vision, mood swings, and unconsciousness. Health problems associated with long-term alcohol consumption are more serious. They include a higher risk for heart and liver disease, circulatory problems, peptic ulcers, irreversible brain damage, and various forms of cancer.

- TRANS-FATS—HYDROGENATED FATS

Trans-fats were invented by scientists so that liquid oils could be "hydrogenated" and have a longer shelf life. They are really bad fats that turn into life-destroying free radicals in the body, and they should always be avoided. Trans-fats fill up all the "fat spaces" in our cells, much like cars take up parking spaces—they are especially dangerous because they are impossible for the body to absorb, and they make it impossible for good fats to be absorbed. Trans-fats are found in many commercially-packaged foods including french fries, microwave popcorn, vegetable shortening, and stick margarine.

- FRIED FOODS

In April of 2002, a team of Swedish researchers discovered that fried foods contain a potentially cancer-causing (carcinogenic) chemical called acrylamide. Acrylamide is formed during traditional cooking such as frying, baking, and roasting. Acrylamide is found in many high-carbohydrate foods that have been manufactured or cooked at high temperatures, including french fries and potato chips. Fried foods offer absolutely no nutritional benefits, and they are readily attributed to health problems.

- DOGHNUTS AND PASTRIES

Fried doughnuts contain about 35 to 40 percent trans-fats. Just to show you how backwards the American health system is, in 2009, a Florida doctor, Jason Newsom, lost his job for publicly speaking out against fried foods. Dr. Newsom worked for the county public health department and was fired for flashing messages on an electronic sign outside his office that said things like "Donuts = Diabetes," "America Dies on Dunkin," "Hamburger = Spare Tire," and "French Fries = Thunder Thighs." In a country where the majority of health care dollars are spent treating diet-related chronic diseases such as cancer, diabetes, and heart disease, this is pretty sad!

• "HEART-HEALTHY" BUTTER SPREADS AND SPRAYS
The human body was not made from chemicals in a lab; and, consequently, it does not recognize fake foods created in labs or foods that have been significantly altered with chemicals and preservatives as food.

The main problem with fake butter (and fake food in general) is that one-half of all of the carbon molecules in it are unattached and indigestible; and so they turn into harmful free radicals that float around in your colon, blood, and lymphatic system and destroy your health. Imitation butter and butter sprays are chemically produced, which means even though they are advertised as heart-healthy, they are definitely not good for your heart or any other part of your body!

As far as real butter goes, your body is a creation of God, and it recognizes other unaltered creations of God (such as animals and plants) as food. This means that when you eat real food, your body knows exactly what to do with it and is able to easily absorb and digest it. So while organic butter might not be an ideal food, and there are some problems with the overconsumption of it, at least it is God-made and the body can digest it. Real butter is a lot healthier than fake butter.

• THE DEADLY WHITES
White sugar, flour, rice, and salt have all been altered to the point that they're void of nutrients and toxic to the body. They have been stripped and bleached till they no longer bear any resemblance to the original substances God created. White sugar is so concentrated and changed from its original form that it's harmful and very addictive. White flour is a gunky, non-nutritious, and cancer-causing substance that immobilizes

immune function. A bleaching agent similar to Clorox makes "bleached" flour white and coal-tar-derived vitamins and minerals known to be carcinogenic are what "enhance" it. White rice is a starchy and non-nutritive, blood-sugar-level spiking carbohydrate, and white "table salt" (iodized), or sodium chloride, is an inorganic compound known to be extremely poisonous to the body. If you are concerned about your health, switch over and only buy and eat unaltered forms of sugar, flour, rice, and salt. Read labels and look for 100% whole wheat bread with no trans-fats or high fructose corn syrup.

● SUGAR AND SUGAR-FREE SWEETENERS
Sugar is a powerful and highly-addictive drug that's at the root of almost all health problems. It feeds Candida yeast and causes fat-storing insulin and triglycerides to spike, and it increases age-accelerating molecules and causes unattractive things like excess weight, excessive sagging and wrinkling, and poor eyesight. Sugar and artificial sweeteners are in almost all processed foods. Artificial sweeteners, including high-fructose corn syrup, are even more harmful and hard on the body than sugar is. Safer sweeteners, like pure maple syrup, dates, raw honey, raw agave nectar, xylitol, and Stevia, should still be limited.

● SOY
Many studies have shown that soy is actually quite harmful to the human body, especially if it's been genetically modified or processed, which in America is almost always the case. All soy beans contain high levels of phytic acid, which reduces the assimilation of calcium, magnesium, copper, iron, and zinc and increases the body's requirement for vitamins D and B12. Textured vegetable protein and soy protein isolate are not good sources of protein because high temperature process-

ing denatures and destroys fragile proteins. Even in their "non GMO" (unaltered) form, soy beans contain potent enzyme inhibitors that are known to cause intestinal problems as well as growth retardation and cancer. All soy contains phytoestrogens which are known to disrupt endocrine function and cause breast cancer and infertility in adult women. Phytoestrogens are potent anti-thyroid agents known to cause hypothyroidism and thyroid cancer. The consumption of soy formula has been linked to autoimmune thyroid disease in infants.

Soy contains high levels of aluminum, which is toxic to the nervous system and kidneys and is linked to Alzheimer's. In addition, soy contains trypsin inhibitors, which interfere with protein digestion and are known to cause pancreatic disorders. When test animals were fed soy containing trypsin inhibitors, they experienced stunted growth. Coincidentally, growth problems have been linked to children fed diets high in phytic acid. Soy has also been linked to infertility in men, particularly those who have eaten it throughout their growing up years.

- DAIRY
Contrary to popular belief, cow's milk, whether it's organic or not, is an impure fluid that was simply intended to feed and nourish baby cows and not humans. When it's consumed regularly, cow's milk has a cumulative negative effect on the human body. In fact, a controlled study of 78,000 nurses done over a twelve-year period revealed that those with the highest dairy consumption didn't have stronger bones at all but actually had the highest rate of osteoporosis! (Google "milk study done on 78,000 nurses.") Not only does milk cause rather than prevent weak bones, it contains scores of active hormones and allergens, cholesterol and fat, antibiotics, and anything the cow has eaten, including weeds and chemical residues from toxic sprays (measurable amounts of herbi-

cides, pesticides, antibiotics, blood, puss, feces, bacteria, and viruses).

Cheese, ice cream, and butter are even more harmful to the body than milk because they contain concentrated amounts of all the bad stuff that's in milk. For instance, it takes ten pounds of milk to make one pound of cheese, which means you get ten times more saturated fat in one bite of cheese than you do in one sip of milk. And you get twelve times more fat in ice cream and twenty-one times more fat in butter. Then there's the matter of homogenizing and pasteurizing milk, which makes milk and other dairy products even less compatible with the human body.

Dairy products are known to cause excess mucus, allergies, eczema, asthma, diabetes, cancer, heart disease, bronchial and pulmonary disease, and digestive problems—including an overgrowth of Candida yeast. If you're going to eat meat and dairy, it is suggested that you, at least, buy grass-fed (better than grain) hormone- and antibiotic-free products from a source you can trust. (FYI—Hormone- and antibiotic-free products can still contain up to 10 percent hormones and antibiotics)

Whey is a dairy product, and good-quality life-culture yogurt and keifer are exceptions to dairy because they have been fermented and can actually be health promoting. Goat's milk, coconut milk, rice milk, almond milk, and oat milk are all much safer and healthier alternatives to cow's milk and soy products. (See Food, Inc. (www.foodincmovie.com) to see what's happening in the meat and dairy industry.)

● MEAT AND PROCESSED MEATS
Most of the meat that's sold in grocery stores and restaurants is loaded with saturated fat, antibiotics, hormones, pesticides, and toxins. Many studies have shown that eating meat (and

dairy products) on a regular basis has a negative cumulative effect on the body. After performing an intensive study on nutrition, Dr. T. Colin Campbell, who is the director of the Division of Nutritional Sciences at Cornell University and former senior advisor to the American Institute for Cancer Research, said, "There is a strong correlation between dietary protein intake and cancer of the breast, prostate, pancreas, and colon." According to this study, animal protein is behind many of the most prevalent and deadly diseases of our time. Results showed that people who derive 70 percent of their protein from animal products have major health difficulties, compared to people who derive just 5 percent of their protein from animal sources. It's a fact that meat consumers have 17 times the death rate from heart disease, and female meat consumers are 5 times more likely to die of breast cancer. Processed meats, including canned meats, hot dogs, and luncheon meats, etc. are the worst because they contain unhealthy additives, cancerous sodium nitrates, and highly processed meat "byproducts." It's always a good idea to stay away from foods with mysterious unnamed ingredients!

When you consider how fat and sick so many people in their teens and 20s are today, you can bet those numbers will get far worse, and at earlier ages, in the very near future. And all of them will be riding around in scooter chairs, parking in handicapped spots and crying about their "disabilities" over pizzas and Big Macs. The next crisis won't be too many sick people—it'll be too few healthy people to care for them.
William Douglass, MD

CLEANSING

The difference between 99% raw and 100% raw is 1,000%!
Anonymous

Regular fasting, meaning the total abstinence from food and water for short periods of time, is good for the entire body because it gives it a boost and helps keep the digestive tract cleaned out and healthy. Typically, this type of fasting is not considered a cleanse though. Controlled fasting, wherein only herbal tea and raw fruit or vegetable juices are consumed for days, is what this book refers to as a "cleanse." During a cleanse, it's typical to drink juices and lots of water and also to take specific herbal supplements.

Periodic cleanses are great for healing and nourishing the body and mind; but if you are seriously toxic, your body might be too weak to handle it. Even if you need major cleansing, you might be in too bad a shape to jump right in. It's very possible that you'll need to prepare your body first. A good way to gently cleanse your body and nourish your liver and restore proper pH balance at the same time is to drink a cup of lemon tea first thing each morning. To make the tea, juice half a lemon and add it to warm water—or use 3–4 drops of lemon essential oil. Wait at least 20 minutes after drinking lemon tea before eating breakfast.

If you've been used to eating a lot of processed foods (sugar, soft drinks/energy drinks, meat, and dairy, etc.) or taking a lot of medicine, switching over to a healthier lifestyle (including taking herbs and essential oils) can cause your body to detox, and initially it can make you feel much worse instead of better. Make sure that you're supporting yourself by drinking plenty of pure water (distilled or oxygenated—one half to three quarters of your body weight in ounces), taking high-quality supplements, exercising (walking and yoga are great), and getting extra rest if you feel like you need to. Doing these things will help prevent an unpleasant "healing crisis."

THE MASTER (LEMONADE) CLEANSE
1/4 cup lemon juice
1/4 cup pure maple syrup
1/4 tsp–3 tsp cayenne (or more)
1 quart pure water (distilled or alkaline)

This cleanse was developed by Stanley Burroughs, and it's a great way to do a cleansing fast. The lemon acts as a purifier and toner, the cayenne increases the circulation, and the maple syrup supplies the necessary glucose to keep energy levels up. Drink one gallon of lemonade a day, along with herbal teas and water— and no food. This cleanse is great for cleansing and rejuvenating the liver.

The Master Cleanse is perfectly safe to do for several days at a time. I know because I did it without cheating for eleven days! The first two days were hard, but then it became easy. In fact, I had increased energy and wasn't at all hungry until the last day. When I woke up feeling like I was starving, I knew I'd cleansed enough and needed to start eating again. And so I did. After this fast, stick with simple, clean foods at first; drink fresh juices, and eat raw green salads, fruits, and broths; and avoid bread, dairy, meat, and sugar.

CHLOROPHYLL-WATER
Chlorophyll water is green and looks like "swamp water." However, it's just pure water with liquid chlorophyll water added to it, and it's actually pretty good—kind of minty tasting. Chlorophyll is a powerful antioxidant that neutralizes free radicals and limits oxidative damage. It is excellent for draw-

ing toxins from the blood and improving blood-cell health. Chlorophyll also nourishes the colon (reduces gassiness) and increases energy levels. To make green water (it's minty tasting), add 1–2 tablespoons of liquid chlorophyll to a gallon of water (distilled is good). Drink it throughout the day.

SLUDGE DRINK—COLON CLEANSE
2 TBS whole leaf aloe
2 TBS chlorophyll
1 TBS hydrated bentonite clay
2 TBS psyllium hulls—powder
1–1 1/2 cups raw, unprocessed apple juice (if you have a juicer, juice apples)
2 cascara sagrada or LBS II (Nature's Sunshine)

Combine all ingredients, except cascara sagrada or LBS II, in a blender. Mix together, and drink quickly before the phyllium becomes gelatinous. Chase with cascara sagrada or LBS II and a big glass of pure water. Sludge drink is great for people with sluggish colons. It can be taken daily, and it does not cause diarrhea.

Substances such as artificial colors, sweeteners, stabilizers, nitrates, and preservatives are often linked to cancer in lab animals and may be harmful or cancer promoting in humans. They are best avoided. You can find out what additives are in a given food by knowing how to read the label.
Dr. Joel Fuhrman

HEALING REAL FOODS

Any time you eat anything other than fruits and vegetables you're eating food for some other reason than nutrition— you're eating it for entertainment, for social value, to numb yourself or because you're addicted to it. Dr. Douglas Graham

Many of the so-called foods Americans think are making them healthy are, in fact, actually wearing down their bodies. Soy, meat, milk (dairy), processed foods (including vitamin and mineral fortified), white sugar and flour, iodized salt, and canned foods, for example, all contribute to poor health. On top of that, there are many harmful chemicals and dyes used in packaging.

For example, Bisphenol-A or BPA, which is readily found in plastic food containers and water bottles, is linked to cancer. (Glass and aluminum water bottles are safe.) And Clorox, which we use to disinfect water, counters, containers, and even fruit and vegetables, is also known to cause cancer. (White vinegar is a natural disinfectant that is safe).

Did you know that most big food suppliers are owned by Monsanto, which is a huge conglomerate that's main concern is controlling the world's food supply?

Monsanto began introducing GMO foods in 1996. In case you don't know about GMO (GE/GM) foods, they are foods that have been genetically modified. Their DNA has been altered through genetic engineering to make them drought tolerant and pest and disease resistant and able to ripen faster. The problem with GMO foods is that up to 5 percent of their DNA spontaneously mutates in unpredictable ways.

In a study done in the early 1990s, rats were force-fed genetically modified tomatoes after they refused to eat them on their own (animals repeatedly turn their nose up at GMO foods). After the rats ate the GMO tomatoes, several of them developed stomach lesions; and within two weeks, seven out of forty died. And yet, the tomatoes were approved by the FDA. This is just one of many studies that have shown GMO foods to be very harmful. Food allergies, digestive problems, behavior disorders, stunted growth, infertility, and early deaths, as well as crop failure, have all been strongly linked to GMO foods. (Google "FDA approved GE tomatoes that killed rats," and "Wisconsin school experiments with mice and GMO food.")

It's sobering to note that almost all of the corn, soy, canola, and sugar grown in the U.S. are GMO crops. (See the documentary movie Food, Inc. to understand the serious and wide-reaching ramifications!)

This means that candy and almost all processed foods (cheap foods) contain one or more GMO ingredients. Also, commercially grown tomatoes and cantaloupes are typically GMO.

Identifying non-GMO produce can be tricky. Fruit is the easiest to identify. Look at the sticker on fruit because there is a PLU code with either 4 or 5 numbers on it. If a fruit's label has 4 numbers, it means it has been conventionally grown and may contain pesticides, but at least isn't GMO. Codes that have five numbers and start with 9 mean the fruit was organically grown and is GMO and pesticide-free. A code that has 5 numbers and starts with 8 means the fruit has been genetically engineered. AVOID all produce with 5 number codes that start with 8. Companies that sell non-GMO foods are beginning to label them as such, so look for GMO symbols on labels. (There's a current push to eliminate labels and make GMO foods a standard).

Not only do you have to look for certified organic and non-GMO stickers and labels, you can't automatically assume that food sold in health-food stores is healthy either, because a lot of it isn't. Before you buy anything that's packaged, read the label and stick with short lists of ingredients that contain words you can pronounce. Always avoid soy and high fructose corn syrup!

All that being said… non-altered and non-sprayed God-made "real" foods do contain many cancer-fighting and health-increasing benefits. And if you are trying to cure cancer or just want to prevent it, and also like the idea of feeling and looking your best, there's nothing like fresh and wholesome real foods to nourish your body, put a spring in your step, and give you a radiant healthy glow!

As much as possible, grow your own food (use heirloom seeds), or buy locally-grown fresh produce from an organic farmer or a source you know and can trust. In case you think high-quality organic fruits and vegetables are too expensive, just consider the long-term cost of eating cheap junk food. (It's a sad fact that statistics show 90 percent of a typical American's food budget is spent on fast food or processed foods—no wonder so many people have deadly diseases!)

In case you're worried about the cost of eating organic produce, keep in mind that when your body is getting the nutrients it needs (instead of a lot of harmful fillers), it won't require nearly as much food, and you'll be satisfied with eating less.

Many of the following fruits, vegetables, grains, and nuts are actually quite inexpensive, especially when they're in season; and they're all super nutritious.

• APPLES
Apples skins contain antioxidants and fiber. They are high in pectin, which is a soluble fiber that helps reduce high cholesterol. Apples have been shown to help ward off obesity, diabetes, lung and heart disease, and cancer. For the most health benefits, make sure you buy organic apples and eat them raw—and leave the skin on.

● APRICOTS

Apricots are rich in beta carotene, which helps prevent free-radical damage and protect the eyes. The body turns beta-carotene into Vitamin A, which may help ward off some cancers, especially of the skin. Eat apricots fresh when they are in season. When they aren't in season, eat unsweetened dried apricots.

● ASPARAGUS

Asparagus is a natural laxative and diuretic that contains folic acid, potassium, phosphorous, iron, copper, zinc, and vitamins C and B. Asparagus also contains high levels of folate, which is essential for healthy heart function, and glutathione. Glutathione is a powerful antioxidant that supports immune health and brain function. In studies, glutathione has been shown to protect against at least thirty carcinogens.

● AVACADOS

Avocados are loaded with oleic acid, which is a good type of fat that lowers cholesterol. They contain significant amounts of beta-sitosterol, which lowers blood cholesterol; potassium, which regulates blood pressure; and folate, which is good for heart health. Avocados also contain generous amounts of vitamin K, vitamin B6, vitamin C, copper, and fiber—which is why they say that an avocado a day keeps the doctor away!

● BANANAS

Bananas contain high levels of potassium and decent amounts of other vitamins and minerals. They have been shown to have antibiotic properties. Bananas soothe the stomach and strengthen the stomach lining against acids and ulcers, and they regulate blood pressure.

- BARLEY

Barley is rich in fiber, selenium, niacin, and antioxidants that protect against cancer. Barley offers good protection against high blood pressure, heart disease, and type 2 diabetes. Make sure to buy un-hulled barley and not the polished type.

- BEANS

Beans contain generous amounts of high-quality protein, fiber, and nutritious fat. They reduce high cholesterol and protect against obesity, diabetes, and heart disease. Many studies have shown that beans inhibit cancerous growth in normal cells and reduce the risk of getting cancer in the first place.

- BERRIES

Berries are low in calories and high in fiber, and they're loaded with plant compounds that improve memory and fight cancer. All berries are excellent sources of fiber, vitamin C, and phyto-nutrients (polyphenols), which strengthen the immune system. Berries offer vitally important antioxidant protection. Blueberries, in particular, are very beneficial in fighting disease.

- BROCCOLI (AND CAULIFLOWER)

Broccoli and cauliflower contain high amounts of vitamins, fiber, and antioxidants. Broccoli is rich in carotene, vitamin C, and quercetin, and it helps prevent ulcers. Cauliflower contains high levels of vitamin C, folate, and cancer-fighting photonutrients. Both broccoli and cauliflower are known to be effective in helping prevent lung, colon, and breast cancer.

- CABBAGE

Cabbage contains numerous antioxidant and anticancer compounds. It is rich in vitamin C, beta carotene, folic acid, and fiber. Cabbage suppresses the growth of colon polyps, which are a precursor to colon cancer. Studies have shown that eating cabbage more than once a week significantly decreases the chance of getting colon-cancer.

- CANTALOUPES
Cantaloupes contain vitamin C (almost twice the recommended daily dose in half a melon) and beta-carotene, which are both powerful antioxidants that help protect cells from free-radical damage. Half of a melon contains almost twice as much potassium as a banana does, which also helps lower blood pressure.

- CARROTS
Carrots contain very high amounts of beta-carotene which is known to prevent numerous health problems, including heart attacks, cataracts, and cancer. One study showed that by simply eating one cup of raw carrots a day, a person can significantly decrease his or her risk of strokes, heart attacks, and lung cancer.

- CELERY
Celery provides an excellent source of vitamin C and fiber, as well as folic acid, potassium, calcium, and vitamins B1, B6, and B2. Celery contains phytochemical compounds known as coumarins, which have been shown to be effective in cancer prevention. Due to the high levels of potassium and sodium, fresh celery-based juices are great electrolyte-replacement drinks. Celery is a good natural diuretic that helps the body rid itself of toxins.

- CHIA SEEDS
Chia seeds are good sources of calcium, phosphorus, magnesium, manganese, copper, niacin, zinc, and soluble fiber.

Chia seeds have approximately three times to ten times the healthy oil concentrations of most grains; they are a rich source of Omega-3 fatty acids. They are also rich in the unsaturated fatty acid linoleic acid, which the body cannot manufacture.

• COCONUTS—THAI COCONUT (COCONUT OIL, MILK, WATER, & CREAM)

Unhydrogenated, unprocessed coconut oil is considered to be one of the healthiest fats. (This is not to be confused with hydrogenated coconut oil, which can be found in processed foods and is very harmful). Unprocessed coconut oil is a significant and rare source of medium-chain fatty acids (MCFAs) and is extremely beneficial to the body. MCFAs can actually increase the efficiency of EFAs by as much as 100 percent. Most foods contain long-chain fatty acids that need pancreatic enzymes and bile to be digested, but medium-chain fatty acids do not. Coconut oil is 64 percent MCFAs, which means that, unlike other fats, it is immediately burned in the body as fat. Because medium-chain triglycerides don't require bile to digest them, many hospitals around the world use coconut oil to treat people with digestion problems.

Coconut oil supplies energy to cells and regulates blood sugar. It improves insulin secretion and the utilization of blood glucose and is very good for diabetics. It purifies the blood and satisfies hunger and helps control sugar cravings. Coconut oil is highly alkaline and known to prevent heart disease and inhibit cancer. Coconut oil is antibacterial, antiviral, anti-parasitic, and anti-fungal. It is beneficial for hypoglycemia, gallbladder problems, osteoporosis, and diseases like chronic fatigue syndrome and Crohn's disease. Coconut oil also contains monolaurin, which helps the body deal with viruses and bacteria-causing diseases such as herpes, influenza, cytomegalovirus, and HIV.

Coconut oil contains large amounts of lauric acid, which is a powerful antimicrobial and immune-function compound that naturally occurs in breast milk. When lauric acid is consumed, it converts up in the form of energy. Most baby formulas contain coconut oil; however, it's not unprocessed coconut oil. Instead, the formulas contain a cheap, processed, and inferior product. You can tell the quality of coconut oil by its flavor; the poorer quality it is, the less flavorful it is. Virgin, unprocessed coconut oil, tastes so good you can eat it by the spoonful. In case you don't know, the liquid inside coconuts is referred to as water or juice. Coconut cream is made from pressing the coconut meat, and coconut milk is made from the expressed juice of grated coconut meat and water. Unprocessed coconut oil and cream can be found in health-food stores. Raw Thai coconuts are one of the most nutritious types of coconut. They are available in many ethnic and health-food markets. (See how to open a Thai coconut at www.greensmoothiegirl.com.)

● COLLARD GREENS
Collard greens are loaded with antioxidant compounds, including lutein, vitamin C, and beta carotene. Collard green consumption (along with other dark leafy greens) is associated with low rates of cancer. Studies done on animals have shown that collared-green consumption inhibits the spread of breast cancer.

● CRANBERRIES
Cranberries are high in nutrients and antioxidant-rich vitamins. They help fight bladder infections by preventing harmful bacteria from growing. Cranberry juice is a popular form of treatment; however, most bottled cranberry juice contains sugar, which actually defeats the purpose. For the most ben-

efits, either juice fresh cranberries (they can be frozen when in season), or buy 100 percent juice without added sugar. Or take sugar-free cranberry pills or capsules.

● DATES
Dates are a high-carbohydrate food that's rich in fiber and packed with fruit sugar, which makes them a healthy natural sweetener. Dates are also high in natural pain relievers (salicylates) and fiber, and they have a laxative effect on the body. Dried fruits, including dates, are linked to lower rates of certain cancers, especially pancreatic cancer.

● EGGPLANT
Eggplants contain calcium, folate, phytonutrients, phenolic compounds, and flavonoids, which are powerful antioxidants that help protect cell membranes and reduce toxins inside the body. Studies suggest that eating eggplant lowers blood cholesterol and helps counteract some of the detrimental effects of high-fat foods. Lab tests also show that eggplant acts as a mild diuretic and antibacterial agent.

● FATS (GOOD)
Good fats play such a vital role in keeping the body healthy and vibrant that I'm clumping them all together (some are also listed singly) and including them in this list of foods to be included in your healthy diet.

Monosaturated fats are the healthiest types of fats because they lower total cholesterol and LDL cholesterol (the bad type) while increasing HDL cholesterol (the good type). Avocados and nuts, including peanuts, walnuts, almonds, and pistachios, and flax and olive oil are high in monounsaturated fats. Make sure to only eat fresh, raw, and unprocessed nuts though, because "sitting" for too long makes nuts and seeds rancid, and "roasting" them turns them into unhealthy fats. The best way to store raw nuts is in the freezer.

When choosing "oils," keep in mind that no matter what the label says, all processed oils are unhealthy. This includes canola, corn, vegetable, safflower, sunflower, soy, cotton-seed, and hydrogenated peanut butter. Canola oil is touted as healthy because it contains linoleic acid (omega-6), but it's also known to contain rapeseed and have negative effects on the body; plus, canola oil is usually a GMO food—so it's best to avoid it. (Google "dangers of canola/rapeseed oil.")

Unprocessed coconut oil, flaxseed oil, and grapeseed oil also contain significant levels of linoleic acid, but they are known to be much more beneficial than canola, corn, or soy, so stick with them.

Keep in mind that just because healthy fats are good for you does not mean it's good to overdo it when eating them. Generally all you need is a couple of tablespoons a day; and one is enough if you're trying to lose weight. You might need more healthy fats if you are malnourished, fat deprived, or trying to gain weight.

Raw nuts, flaxseed oil, coconut oil, olive oil, and avocados are all excellent sources of fats, and one or more should be eaten daily in place of, but not in addition to, unhealthy fats.

• FLAX SEEDS (FLAX OIL)
Flax seeds are rich in essential fatty acids that cannot be manufactured by the body. EFAs are important for making and repairing cell membranes and eliminating waste from the cells. They support many body systems, including the nervous system, immune system, cardiovascular system, and reproductive system and are essential for regulating blood pressure and clotting and maintaining a healthy heart rate. They are essential for fertility and proper neural development.

Flaxseeds are also good sources of linolenic acid (Omega-3), which is important for vital organ function and intracellular activity. Flaxseed oil is available in liquid form or in capsules and is sold in health-food stores. It's good to buy flax oil in smaller bottles, because once it is opened, it will begin to oxidize and go rancid (this is true of all unprocessed oils). When purchasing whole flaxseeds, smell them to make sure they aren't rancid—only buy organic and fresh flaxseeds. Store flaxseeds in the freezer to keep them fresh. Whole flaxseeds pass through the digestive system without breaking down, so they need to be soaked overnight or ground in a coffee grinder just before they are used. Flaxseeds begin to lose their nutritive value once they are ground.

• GARLIC

Garlic has medicinal properties that have been well-known for thousands of years. Hundreds of published studies support garlic's antimicrobial effects as well as its ability to lower the risk of heart disease. It is a proven antibiotic that's been shown to kill bacteria, fungi, and intestinal parasites. It contains multiple antioxidants, immune-system boosters, and anticancer compounds. Garlic is a natural anticoagulant, decongestant, and anti-inflammatory agent. It is known to lower blood-cholesterol levels, and it is a very effective medicine for treating colds.

• GRAPES

Grapes contain vitamins A, B, and C and thirteen minerals, including high doses of potassium and quercetin. Quercetin is a powerful antioxidant, anti-histamine, and anti-inflammatory. Research shows that quercetin may help prevent cancer, especially prostate cancer. The skins of red grapes contain reveratrol, which is a polyphenol that lowers the bad-type of LDL cholesterol.

• HONEY (RAW)

Studies recently done in Japan and Australia showed that people with advanced stages of stomach and bone cancer were successfully cured by taking one tablespoon of raw honey with one teaspoon of cinnamon powder three times a day for one month. Processed honey—the type of honey typically sold in grocery stores—does not offer the same health benefits. Make sure to buy raw, and if possible, locally-grown honey. Raw honey crystalizes, but do not heat it to soften it because high temperatures will destroy its healing properites. Health-food stores often carry local raw honey. (FYI—applying equal parts of raw honey and cinnamon powder over affected skin is known to cure eczema, ringworm, and all types of skin infections).

• KALE

Kale is an ultra-rich source of anticancer compounds and chemicals. Kale contains beta-carotene, lutein, and indoles and can prevent and protect against estrogen-linked cancers, as well as cataracts and macular degeneration.

• MUSHROOMS

Mushrooms contain several important nutrients, including copper, potassium, folate, and niacin. The Reishi mushroom is an excellent immune system booster that's used to treat a wide range of conditions, including heart disease, cancer, and high blood pressure. Shiitake mushrooms are protective antioxidants that build the immune system and inhibit the formation of arteriosclerotic plaque. They are known to help prevent against cardiovascular disease, strokes, and diabetes. Plus they regulate blood clotting and sugar levels and help reduce cholesterol. Reishi and Shitake mushrooms are regarded as powerful heart and cancer-preventative medicine in Asia. In Japan, Shiitake mushrooms are used along with chemotherapy to improve its effectiveness.

● NUTS

Nuts are packed with protein, fiber, monounsaturated fats, vitamin E, folic acid, magnesium, copper, and antioxidants. They help reduce the risks of heart disease, diabetes, and cancer. Even though they contain fat, nuts help control weight. Processed (roasted) nuts won't provide health benefits, so make sure to eat raw nuts.

● OATS

Oats are high in fiber and nutrients, including manganese (which contains essential trace minerals needed for healthy skin, bone, and cartilage formation), selenium (essential trace mineral that protects cells against free radicals), and tryptophan (essential amino acid needed for survival). Many studies have shown that eating a bowl of oatmeal in the morning can help prevent and turn around heart disease and diabetes. Compounds in oats are also thought to help control nicotine cravings.

● OLIVE OIL

Olive oil is a monosaturated fat that breaks down stored fat in the body. It is rich in oleic acid (omega-9), vitamin E, chlorophyll, polyphenols, and carotenoids, which are known to be powerful antioxidants. Studies indicate that people who eat virgin olive oil on a regular basis experience less cancer, heart disease, diabetes, asthma, inflammation, bone loss, and atherosclerosis than people who don't. For the greatest health benefits, use 1–2 tablespoons of extra virgin olive oil a day— but not more, unless you are trying to gain weight.

Olive oil loses much of its healing power when it's heated to high temperatures (it turns into a trans-fat), so eat it raw by drizzling it over salads, steamed vegetables, whole grain breads, and pastas.

• ONIONS

Onions (chives, shallots, scallions, and leeks) are strong antioxidants that fight bacterial and viral infections. Studies show that eating onions regularly heals certain types of cancer. Onions are rich sources of quercetin, which is a potent antioxidant known to inhibit stomach cancer. Onions also raise good HDL cholesterol levels and help prevent atherosclerosis and blood clots.

• PARSLEY (AND CILANTRO)

Parsley is a very nutritious antioxidant herb that's high in vitamin K, which is necessary for proper bone formation, blood clotting, and helping the body transport calcium. Parsley is also a good source of vitamins A, C, and K, beta-carotene, lutein, and zeaxanthin, which help to preserve vision. Parsley contains volatile oils, which have been shown to inhibit the formation of tumors in animals, particularly in the lungs. Parsley is a great detoxifier that rids the body of carcinogens, including those in tobacco smoke. It also acts as a diuretic.

Cilantro, also known as Asian parsley (coriander), is another tasty "garnish herb" that's very rich in antioxidants. Cilantro lowers blood sugar and cholesterol levels and cleanses the body of heavy metals (including from vaccinations).

• PLUMS (PRUNES)

Plums and prunes are good sources of potassium, vitamin A (beta-carotene), B1 (thiamine), B2 (riboflavin), and fiber. They contain compounds that act as antibacterial and antiviral agents, and they can strengthen eyes and help retain good vision. Plums are high in fiber and are good natural laxatives.

• POMEGRANATES

Pomegranates are potassium-rich and considered "superfoods" because of their ultra-high antioxidant properties. Some research suggests that pomegranate juice slows the progression of certain types of cancer and keeps cancers from returning. Other research shows that it reverses hardening of the arteries and lowers blood pressure. Watch out for and avoid pomegranate "flavored" juices.

● POTATOES (HEIRLOOM)
Nutritional analysis done on heirloom varieties of potatoes has shown that homegrown heirloom potatoes are much more nutritious than russet or new potatoes that have been mass produced or grown on huge agribusiness "farms." Not only are farmers who grow heirloom crops far more likely to use organic fertilizers, but the plants themselves are able to absorb more nutrients because they haven't been bred for other purposes. If you have a place to do so, try growing your own organic heirloom potatoes. Even though they tend to be tiny, they are so nutritious and delicious that it makes up for their small size! Both the skin and flesh of heirlooms potatoes are very nutritious.

● PUMPKINS—PUMPKIN SEEDS
Pumpkins contain loads of fiber and "medicinal" nutrients. They are excellent sources of beta-carotene and alpha-carotene, which are associated with reversing aging and protecting against certain types of cancer. Plus pumpkin seeds are one of the most nutritious and medicinal seeds. Pumpkin seeds have anti-inflammatory properties and are known to lower cholesterol, improve prostate health, increase men's bone density, and help rid the body of parasites.

● RICE (BROWN)
Brown rice is far more nutritious than white rice because during the milling process that turns brown rice into white rice,

almost 70 percent of the nutrients are removed. Brown rice is very high in maganese, and it's a good source of selanium, magnesium, and tryptophan. Brown rice has antioxidant and anticancer properties. It can lower cholesterol, prevent kidney stones, promote weight loss, and stop diarrhea.

• SALMON
Salmon is low in calories and saturated fat and high in protein and omega-3 fatty acids, which are necessary for good health. Salmon is a good source of selenium, niacin, vitamins B12 and B6, phosphorus, and magnesium. Eating salmon (and tuna) can help lower triglycerides, control blood pressure, and protect against stroke and heart attack. It can also lower blood sugar levels and decrease inflammation. For the most benefits, eat broiled or baked salmon (not fried), and make sure it comes from clean and fresh water.

• SPINACH
Spinach is a super low-calorie food that's rich in antioxidants, including vitamins A, K, and C, folate, magnese, lutien, beta carotene, magnesium, and iron. Calorie for calorie, spinach (and other leafy green vegetables) provides more nutrients than any other food. Regular consumption of spinach is linked with much lower rates of cancer.

• SWEET POTATOES
Sweet potatoes are rich in antioxidants, including vitamin A and C, beta-carotene, manganese, copper, and fiber. Studies have shown that sweet potatoes increase the antioxidant activity of glutathione, which is one of the body's most impressive internally-produced antioxidants. Glutathione promotes improved immune and brain function.

- SWISS CHARD

Swiss chard is an extremely nutritious "green"; both the leaves and stems are very high in cancer-fighting vitamins and minerals. Swiss chard helps maintain good bone health and mental function. When eaten raw, like in green smoothies, it offers more disease-fighting and healing benefits than almost any other vegetable. Swiss chard protects against emphysema and is a valuable food for smokers (or people who live with smokers).

- TOMATOES

Tomatoes contain lycopene, which is one of the strongest polyphenols or powerful antioxidants. They are also extremely good sources of vitamin C. Research shows that eating tomatoes daily may cut the risk of bladder, stomach, and colon cancers in half. For the most benefits, make sure to buy organic non-GMO tomatoes (GMO are common in commercially-grown tomatoes), and drizzle fresh tomato slices with virgin olive oil—because lycopene is best absorbed when eaten with a little healthy fat.

- WATERMELON

Watermelon is an antioxidant-rich fruit. Watermelons are very concentrated sources of the carotenoid lycopene, and according to research published in the Asia Pacific Journal of Clinical Nutrition (Jian L, Lee AH, et al.), "regularly eating lycopene-rich fruits, such as watermelon, (and drinking green tea) may greatly reduce a man's risk of developing prostate cancer."

- WHEAT (WHEAT GERM AND BRAN)

Whether or not wheat is good for you is a controversial subject, so I will simply tell you the facts as I know them. White flour should always be avoided because it has been stripped and altered to the point that it's actually a poisonous and digestive system–clogging substance. On the other hand, wheat in its natural unrefined non-GMO form contains an impressive array of important nutrients. Whole wheat kernals, wheat germ, and wheat bran are all rich sources of maganese, and they're also high in fiber, triptophan, and magnesium. Wheat has a laxative effect on the body. It has been shown to decrease inflammation, lower the risk of type 2 diabetes, improve gastrointestinal health, prevent gallstones, and reduce the risk of cancer. Unfortunately, wheat has largely become a GMO product, which is why it has become such an irritant. Something else to watch out for in baked goods is high-fructose syrup. This is a very harmful sweetener that's commonly added to processed and baked foods.

Sensitivities to wheat, including algergies, celiac disease, gluten intolerance, and Chron's disease, are commonly caused by genetically-modified wheat (GMO). An overgrowth of Candida yeast in the digestive tract is also known to cause wheat sensitivities. Going on the yeast-free diet and avoiding all wheat (grains), dairy, sugar, and processed foods for an extended period of time will give your gut a break and enable it to heal. Healing can take as long as nine months to a year. Once all Candida yeast has been cleared from your system and your digestive system has recovered, you should be able to slowly reintroduce some wheat and grains into your diet and be just fine.

That said, I am sensitive to wheat, and I do best when I avoid it altogether except when it is sprouted. Sourdough whole wheat bread made from sprouted wheat doesn't bother me a bit. To make it, simply soak untreated wheat for 36 hours (make sure kernals are completely covered with water), and then drain and dry them at 115 degrees in a food dehydrator. Dried dehydrated wheat can then be ground and made into bread as usual. Sourdough is recommended because it's less irritating than yeast bread.

● YOGURT (KEIFER)

Plain yogurt is a fermented dairy product that should not be confused with sweetened convenience-size yogurts, including those claiming to be acidophilus-rich, like Activa. Plain yogurt is a very good source of calcium, phosphorus, riboflavin, vitamin B2, and iodine. It also contains live bacterial cultures that are necessary for fighting harmful Candida yeast and restoring healthy balance to the digestive tract. Eating fermented products like yogurt and keifer has been shown to lower LDL (bad) cholesterol, raise HDL (good) cholesterol, strengthen the immune system, and increase fat loss/lower body fat. It's easy and inexpensive to make high quality yogurt at home once you understand the basics. A good yogurt-making kit is recommended.

NOURISHING & HEALING RAW FOOD DIET

When the blood is clogged up from eating processed foods, oxygen cannot freely flow to all parts of the body. This creates blood sludge. This sludge is caused by eating thick, mucousy, rubbery, fatty foods. This not only compromises oxygen transportation, but creates a constipated, disease-causing colon. When you eat raw foods, the blood begins to purify, and you begin to feel like a different person. Raw veganism is the healthiest dietary regimen known to man. Philip McCoy

When food is heated above 116 degrees F°, its enzymes, minerals, vitamins, and "life-force" are destroyed. For this reason, it is advisable to eat at least 75 percent of your food raw. Live, enzyme-rich food is much more nutritious and easier to digest than cooked food. However, if you're used to eating a diet rich in meat, dairy, sweets, simple carbs, and caffeine, it's likely that in the beginning switching to raw food will make you feel a lot worse instead of better. Hence, you might think that your body can't tolerate raw fruits and vegetables, but actually, they are exactly what it needs to heal! Feeling bad just means you're detoxing. This is essential for healing, so hang in there! Normal detox symptoms include headaches, nausea, fatigue, and extreme cravings (feeling like you're starving!). These symptoms can be severe and extremely unpleasant, and they can last for a week or more.

Switching over to a raw-food diet is worth the initial discomfort it might cause because it will pay off in increased healthy digestion, healthy weight loss, improved skin (more tone and a healthy glow), increased energy, and decreased heart disease, diabetes, cancer, and other diseases.

Raw-food diets are fairly simple because they mainly consist of eating unprocessed and uncooked plant foods, such as fresh fruit and vegetables, sprouts, seeds, nuts, grains, beans, dried fruit, and seaweed (highly nutritious!). If you begin eating raw and find you just can't cut it, don't completely throw in the towel. Slow down, and mainly focus on incorporating more raw foods into your meals. Then try eating raw for one meal a day, and increase up to one or two days a week. Raw organic foods are actually very filling and satisfying; so once you get in the swing of it, it's not that hard to eat raw.

That said, raw food diets don't agree with everyone. This could be explained by the Chinese philosophy that some people have a condition called internal dampness, which stems from a weak spleen. In this case, eating raw, cold foods is much like putting a soggy wet log on an already sputtering fire.

If raw foods really don't agree with you, here are some suggestions for strengthening your spleen, which could very possibly take care of the problem.

• Clean up your diet—avoid damp and accumulating foods such as sugar, dairy, and "bad fats;" greasy, oily, and fatty foods; and foods that are rich, cold, and raw in nature.

- Eat aromatic herbs and spices and yellow/orange foods that support spleen function, such as carrots, pumpkins, squash, sweet potatoes, parsnips, apples, red lentils, cardamom, ginger, garlic, and rice.

- Sit up straight when you eat (don't slump), and chew your food thoroughly—it helps with digestion.

- Don't drink ice water with meals—sipping warm herbal tea is acceptable.

- Exercise regularly—get up and get your body moving every day.

- Stop worrying—overthinking weakens the spleen and creates sluggish digestion; so make it a regular practice to clear your mind with meditation and relaxation breathing.

- Restore your digestive fire—take spleen-strengthening tonic herbs. Also consider acupuncture, acupressure, or Jin Shin Jyutsu treatments.

GREEN SMOOTHIES

When you're green inside, you're clean inside.
Dr. Bernard Jensen

There are lots of very good reasons why you should be making green smoothies and feeding them to your household by the pint- and quart-full every day. Namely, they are the fastest, easiest, and most enjoyable way to get plenty of healthy, raw greens into you and your family! Green smoothies are filling, they taste surprisingly good (really!), and they can be made in minutes and consumed on the run (for adults, pour them into recycled quart-size jars). Green smoothies can slow down aging and help keep you slim and vibrantly beautiful; they can keep you stay healthy so that you may never need to go to the doctor again.

In the beginning, you might need a recipe; but as you get used to making green smoothies, I think you'll find it easy and fun to come up with your own combinations. To start with, you'll need a good blender like a Vita-Mix or Blend-Tec. If you don't have one already, it's an investment worth making.

The main ingredients for a green smoothie are as follow:

• Liquid—distilled or alkalized water, coconut milk, almond milk, rice milk, and/or unsweetened juice (preferably fresh). Or if you're really serious about your health, you can do like I do and use rejuvalac and/or keifer water for the liquid.

• Good quality plant-based protein powder and/or good quality yogurt—this is optional, but I almost always add a scoop of vanilla protein because it makes smoothies more creamy and delicious. My favorite brands of protein powders are Vegan Trim Shake, Green Smoothie Girl, Life's Basics, and Sun Warrior.

• Lots of organic dark-green leafy vegetables—typically as many as will fit in a Blend-Tec or Vita-Mix after you've added everything else. Use any combination of greens or just one green. Greens can include spinach, romaine lettuce, kale, Swiss chard, wheat grass, and unsprayed edible "weeds," such as dandelion, purslane, and lambsquarters. (Washed greens can be frozen and used later.)
• Chunks of fresh or frozen fruit. (Freeze extra chunks of fresh fruit for later use.)

- Sweetener—agave nectar, Stevia, or pitted dates—use more than the recipe calls for if you need to.

- Soaked almonds, coconut oil, and flaxseed oil, or ground flax seeds, chia seeds, etc.—for added nutritional value.

- 1–2 tsp. Redmond or bentonite clay, or food-grade diatomaceous earth—this is optional but very good for healing ulcers and colon problems.

- Ice cubes—optional (can use chunks of frozen fruit).

To make a green smoothie, put all ingredients in a Blend-Tec or Vita-Mix blender. Start with liquid, usually water or water and coconut milk; then add other ingredients and mix well, until smooth. Don't worry about exact amounts, because it doesn't really matter. Add more liquid or sweetener if you need to. Be sure to vary the types of fruit and greens you use daily so that you'll get a variety of nutrients and not run into the "same old, same old" rut. (Just so you know, green smoothies don't always turn out green!)

COCONUT BERRY SMOOTHIE
2 cups chilled coconut milk
1 cup fresh or frozen raspberries
1 cup fresh or frozen strawberries
1 cup good quality plain yogurt
1–2 TBS agave nectar
1 tsp coconut oil
1–2 handfuls spinach
Ice—optional

COCONUT DATE SMOOTHIE
2 cups chilled coconut milk
1 scoop Life's Basics vanilla protein powder
1 TBS coconut oil
2 TBS ground flax seeds
1 tsp pure vanilla extract
1/4 tsp almond extract
4–6 pitted dates
1–2 handfuls Swiss chard, spinach, or kale
Ice cubes—optional

PINAPPLE COCONUT GINGER SMOOTHIE
1–2 cups pure water
1 cup coconut milk or juice
1 cup fresh pineapple chunks or 1/2 cup frozen pineapple
juice concentrate
2 TBS coconut oil
1 banana
1/4–1/2 TBS fresh peeled gingerroot
2 large handful of spinach leaves
Ice cubes—optional

REAL GREEN SMOOTHIE
2 cups pure water
Juice of 1 freshly squeezed lemon
1 large cucumber
1/2 avocado
1–2 TBS Flaxseed oil
Greens to fill blender—kale, Swiss chard, spinach
1 green delicious apple
Dash of real salt
Agave nectar, if desired
Ice cubes—optional

MORNING MOJITO
1 banana or peach
1 apple
3-4 large kale leaves
A few mint leaves
1 cup of pure water (or more)
 4 ice cubes

HEALER'S CHOICE SMOOTHIE
1 cup blackberries
1 bunch parsley
2–3 large kale leaves
3 large carrots
2 pears
3 stalks celery

WHEATGRASS SMOOTHIE
1 cup cold water
1/2 oz. wheatgrass (or barley grass)
Small slice of ginger
1/2 lemon, juiced
1 apple, cored
2 peaches or 1 mango (can be frozen)
1 frozen banana

PURE ENERGY SMOOTHIE
1/2 cup oats (wheat berries or other sprouted grain works too)
1/4 cup any raw nuts or seeds
1 TBS`flax oil
1 cup kefir
1/2 cup unsweetened almond milk (or coconut milk or coconut water)
1 banana
 1 cup frozen blueberries

1–2 handfuls of spinach and/or kale
1 scoop super green food
1/2" piece of fresh ginger (powder works too)
Dash of cinnamon, nutmeg, and vanilla
1TBS local raw honey—optional (can also sweeten with dates or stevia)

CLASSIC YUMMY SMOOTHIE
3 cups water
2 dates, or a big squirt of agave nectar
1/4 cup soaked almonds
1 TBS ground flaxseeds (or flaxseed oil)
1 TBS chia seeds
1 scoop Life's Basics plant protein powder
1 TBS coconut oil
1 cup frozen blueberries
1 large handful Swiss chard leaves
1 large kale leaf
1 large handful spinach leaves
1 banana, or frozen banana pieces (optional)
Ice (optional)

Put ingredients in a Vita-Mix or Blend-Tec blender, and blend well.

I have never known anyone in 20 years to metastasize or affect another secondary area after the enzymes were started.
Dr. Pierce N.D.

JUICING

There's no trick to juicing; you just wash your organic fruits and veggies well. Then chop them in small enough pieces to fit in the chopper, and run them through a juicer. You don't usually need to peel anything that's organic; but if your fruits and vegetables are not organic, make sure to peel them or scrub them well with a veggie-wash spray.

Although there are many juice recipes available, you can easily come up with your own delicious combinations. If you're making more than a glassful, try collecting the juice in a glass and then pouring it into a pitcher and mixing everything together before drinking.

Fresh juices usually contain high concentrations of natural sugars that cause blood-sugar levels to spike significantly, so make sure to dilute freshly squeezed juice with equal amounts of water (or drink water immediately after drinking the juice). For best results, drink fresh juice within a few hours of making it.

BODY CLEANSING SHAKE
1 cucumber
3 stalks celery
1 beet
3–4 carrots
1 clove garlic
Handful of parsley

VEGGIE DELITE
1/2 tomato
1/4 cucumber
1 carrot
1 celery stalk

1 handful spinach
1/2 red pepper
1/2 cup cabbage
1 green onion
Unprocessed sea salt and pepper

BLUSHING BEAUTY
5 carrots
1 apple
1/2 beet
1 piece of ginger root

RISE AND SHINE
2 pears
3 pink grapefruit
1 sweet potato

MORNING GLORY
3 oranges
2 hard pears
1 small sweet potato

ORANGE GINGER SPRITZER
6 oranges
About 1/2 inch slice ginger root
1/2 cup raspberries or strawberries
Juice oranges in a citrus juicer; then mix in a blender with
ginger and berries.

*Your food determines in a large measure how
long you shall live—how much you shall enjoy life, and how
successful your life shall be.* Dr. Kirschner

WHY PH MATTERS

One must not forget that recovery is brought about
not by the physician, but by the sick man himself. He heals
himself, by his own power, exactly as he walks by means
of his own power, or eats, or thinks, breathes or sleeps.
Georg Groddeck, 1923

When the body performs optimally, the way it was designed
to, that's a sign that it is vibrantly healthy. Vibrant health is
so much more than just looking good or not being sick; it's
having an excess of energy, a clear mind, and a radiant glow.
Obviously this is an optimal state of being!

Vibrant health starts with a proper pH, and that's why it's
super important to keep your pH at an ideal level! The pH of
your body's tissues and fluids determines the levels of your
inner cleanliness or filth—much like it is with a fish tank.
When the water that fish swim in gets too polluted (pH is off),
the fish get sick and die. Just as the correct pH of water is
central to the health and survival of fish, the human body also
needs the right pH in order for us to thrive.

The pH scale is like a thermometer that shows increases and
decreases in the acid and alkaline content of the body's fluids.
A correct pH in the body sets the stage for about 75 trillion cells
to flourish and thrive. The ideal pH is 7.35—7.45. The closer
our body is to that, the higher our level of health and well-being
and the more resistant we are to illness and disease.

When the body's pH is too high or too low, it cannot rid
itself of excess acids and is forced to store them within its
extra-cellular fluids and connective tissue. When this happens
for an extended length of time, cellular integrity is greatly
compromised, and it is inevitable that health problems will
start showing up.

Wellness Made Simple

As you familiarize yourself with the pH of different foods, keep in mind that a food's acid or alkaline-forming tendency in the body has nothing to do with the actual pH of the food itself. For example, lemons are very acidic; but after they are digested and assimilated, they end up being alkaline—which is why lemons are considered very alkaline foods. Meats, on the other hand, are alkaline before they are digested; but they leave very acidic residue in the body. Like nearly all animal products, including dairy, meat is very acid forming and considered an acidic food.

Dark green and bright orange raw vegetables and alkalized water (like Kangen water) create the most alkaline and favorable conditions in the body. Laboratory-produced fake-foods, including microwaved foods, sodas, etc., are all very acidic and harmful and should be avoided as much as possible.

The more acidic you are, the more yeasty you are. You can test your pH with testing strips sold at drug stores. Also, try this easy way to tell if you have yeast: Rinse a clean clear glass with white vinegar and then with distilled water (kills germs); then fill the glass with distilled water, and spit a big amount of saliva into it. Watch what happens. If white streamers start moving down from the spit, you have overgrown yeast.

But today in the United States, and this shows you where fascism REALLY exists, ANY doctor in the United States who cures cancer using alternative methods will be destroyed. You cannot name me a doctor doing well with cancer using alternative therapies that is not under attack. And I KNOW these people; I've interviewed them. Gary Null

PH OF FOODS

Every time you go through a drive-through to eat, you are paying someone to kill you! Anonymous

It is important that you strive to maintain the correct pH, because diseases cannot grow or live in alkaline conditions; but an acidic body is a literal breeding ground for decay and disease. As a rule of thumb, slightly bitter foods tend to be more alkaline, while overly sweet foods tend to be more acidic.

MOST ALKALINE
• Stevia • Lemons • Limes • Grapefruit • Watermelon • Mangoes • Papayas • Asparagus • Onions • Raw vegetable juices • Parsley • Raw spinach • Broccoli • Garlic • Olive oil • Coconut oil • Herbal teas • Lemon water (add fresh lemon juice or pure lemon essential oil) • Oxygenated, alkalized water (like Kangen water)

ALKALINE
• Xylitol • Maple syrup (pure) • Rice syrup • Dates • Figs • Melons • Grapes • Papaya • Kiwi • Berries • Apples • Pears • Raisins • Okra • Squash • Green beans • Beets • Celery • Lettuce (dark) • Zucchini • Sweet potato • Carob • Almonds • Flaxseed oil • Breast milk • Green tea

SLIGHTLY ALKALINE
• Agave nectar • Raw honey • Raw sugar • Oranges • Bananas • Cherries • Pineapple • Peaches • Avocados • Carrots • Tomatoes • Fresh corn • Mushrooms • Cabbage • Peas • Potato skins • Olives • Soybeans • Tofu • Chestnuts • Amaranth • Millet • Wild rice • Quinoa • Soy Milk • Goat's milk • Goat cheese • Whey • Ginger tea

SLIGHTLY ACIDIC

• Processed honey • Molasses • Plums • Processed fruit juices • Cooked spinach • Kidney beans • String beans • Pumpkin seeds • Sunflower seeds • Corn oil • Sprouted wheat bread • Spelt • Brown rice • Eggs • Butter • Yogurt • Buttermilk • Cottage cheese • Black tea • Dark chocolate or cacao nibs (unprocessed chocolate)

ACIDIC

• White sugar • Brown sugar • Sour cherries • Rhubarb • Potatoes (without skins) • Pinto beans • Navy beans • Lima beans • Pecans • Cashews • White rice • Corn • Buckwheat • Oats • Rye • Turkey • Chicken • Lamb • Raw milk • Coffee

MOST ACIDIC

• NutraSweet • Equal • Aspartame • Sweet 'N Low (and other chemical sweeteners) • Blueberries • Cranberries • Prunes • Milk chocolate • Peanuts • Walnuts • Wheat • White flour • Pastries • Fried foods • Pasta • Beef • Pork • Processed meats • Shellfish • Cheese • Pasteurized and homogenized milk, etc. • Ice cream • Beer • Soft drinks • Energy drinks • Sugar-free drinks, such as Crystal Light, etc. • Sports drinks, such as Gatorade and Powerade • Processed foods • Microwaved foods

We are all dietetic sinners; only a small percent of what we eat nourishes us; the balance goes to waste and loss of energy.
William Osler

HOW TO TELL IF YOU HAVE CANDIDA YEAST

You can test your pH with testing strips sold at drug stores. Or another easy and fun way to tell if you have yeast (and are acidic) is to wipe the inside of a clean clear glass with white vinegar and then rinse it with distilled water. This will kill any germs that are on the glass. Next fill the glass with distilled water and spit a big amount of saliva into it, and then watch what happens. If white streamers start moving down from the spit, you will know you have overgrown yeast… and it would be in your best interest to do something about it! Keep in mind that the more acidic you are, the more yeasty you are or the more prolific Candida yeast is in your body.

BAKING SODA pH FIX

Sodium bicarbonate is the time honored method to "speed up" the return of the body's bicarbonate levels to normal. Bicarbonate is inorganic, very alkaline and like other mineral type substances, supports an extensive list of biological functions.
Dr. Mark Sircus, Winning the War on Cancer

Baking soda, also known as sodium bicarbonate, is derived from a natural-occurring mineral. It is known to be a safe and very effective household cleaner, tooth cleaner, and antiperspirant. Baking soda also has strong medicinal properties that make it excellent for healing sunburns and diseases—including cancer! This is probably due to the fact that when baking soda is taken internally, it balances the body's pH and dissolves mucus and soothes mucus membranes.

In 1924, Arm and Hammer published a little book titled "Arm and Hammer Baking Soda Medical Uses," in which a prominent physician, Dr. Volney S. Cheney, stated the following:

"In 1918 and 1919, while fighting the 'flu' with the U. S. Public Health Service, it was brought to my attention that rarely anyone who had been thoroughly alkalinized with bicarbonate of soda contracted the disease, and those who did contract it, if alkalinized early, would invariably have mild attacks."

(FYI—Arm and Hammer Baking Soda contains aluminum, and, therefore, should not be used for healing purposes. Bob's Red Mill Baking Soda, for one, does not contain aluminum. Look for aluminum-free baking soda online.)
     The following healing recipe is from the Arm and Hammer Company in 1925.

RECOMMENDED DOSES FOR COLD AND FLU SYMPTOMS

DAY 1—Take six doses of 1/2 teaspoon of baking soda in a glass of cool water at about two hour intervals.

DAY 2—Take four doses of 1/2 teaspoon of baking soda in a glass of cool water at about two hour intervals.

DAY 3—Take two doses of 1/2 teaspoon of baking soda in a glass of cool water morning and evening. Thereafter, take 1/2 teaspoon in a glass of cool water each morning until cold symptoms are gone.

To take baking soda, dissolve it in a glass of cool water and drink it. More recommendations and instructions for taking sodium bicarbonate can be found in Mark Sircus' book, Sodium Bicarbonate—Rich Man's Poor Man's Cancer Treatment (www.winningcancer.com).

Just so you know, natural substances (including baking soda) are unregulated and cannot be patented, so there is absolutely no money to be made in using them to treat disease, which is why the medical community, as a whole, continues to downplay their worth. In fact, the FDA will no longer allow companies that sell products to make medical claims about them unless they have been tested at great expense and then approved as a drug. This explains why the medical industry and other vested interested groups repeatedly attempt to discredit and destroy doctors and scientists who are speaking out and educating people about inexpensive natural options known to cure cancer and other diseases.

WHY GO ON A YEAST-FREE DIET

It seems that some consideration should be given to the cause of our mounting physical disabilities, but instead of going to the root of our troubles—wrong habits of eating and drinking—we rush to the medicine shelf and smother our uncomfortable and distressing symptoms under an avalanche of pills, potions, and palliatives. Lester Roloff

Candida (Candida albicans) is one of the many micro-organisms/parasites that naturally live in the digestive tract. In a healthy digestive tract, there is a ratio of one yeast cell (harmful bacteria) per million probiotic cells (beneficial bacteria). Under this properly balanced condition, Candida has to fight to survive. But when the body's immune system becomes impaired, or the intestinal pH becomes too acidic, it creates a perfect environment for yeast to grow and thrive, and candidiasis results. Candidiasis is overgrown yeast, or, in other words, it's a state of having more harmful bacteria than beneficial bacteria in the digestive tract.

The digestive tract is lined with a protective mucus membrane that is damaged by candidiasis. When yeast becomes prolific, it changes from a yeast form to a fungal form that grows roots that excrete acid. The acidic roots can then puncture the mucus lining and cause bacteria, yeast, toxins, undigested food particles, and fecal matter to pass through into the bloodstream. This condition, which is often referred to as leaky gut syndrome, is harmful to the body and can make a person very ill. Many people unknowingly suffer from candidiasis and leaky gut syndrome, which is also a result of adrenal burn-out. Prescription medicine doesn't cure candidiasis and leaky gut syndrome or the symptoms caused by them; rather, it only adds fuel to the fire and makes the condition much worse.

The only way to effectively get rid of Candida is to starve it off (hence, the strict version of the yeast-free diet). The unpleasant effects of "die off" are aching, feeling like you're starving, and feeling sick, nauseous, gassy, and bloated. Fortunately, die off is usually short lived. Stay focused on the fact that discomfort means you are winning the war and the yeast is going away! (Due to high stress levels and poor eating habits, just about all Americans have yeast and would benefit from the YF diet.)

THE YEAST-FREE DIET (STRICT)

Along with the strict yeast-free diet, it is highly recommended that you do a Candida cleanse.

TIPS
• Follow the strict version of the yeast-free diet for a two to three week period with absolutely no cheating—cheating will cause you to have huge setbacks! If you have a serious case of yeast, including cancer, it would be good to stay on this strict diet for a month.

- While on the diet, you'll need to restore the proper pH balance in your body. Drinking alkaline water is highly recommended because it neutralizes waste acids. If you can't get alkaline water, at least make sure you are drinking water that is free of fluoride and chlorine—both fluoride and chlorine are known carcinogens.

- While on the diet, make sure you are eating a minimum of 5 veggie servings per day. It's recommended that you add Ultimate Green Zone from Nature's Sunshine to smoothies.

FOODS YOU CAN'T EAT
- No grains of any kind, including corn, rice, Ezekiel bread, and usually oatmeal
- No cooked starchy veggies (carrots, potatoes w/white flesh, peas, corn)
- No vinegar
- No mushrooms
- No dairy (if you are a A, AB, or B blood-type, you might be able to have a little good quality non-sweetened yogurt such as Brown Cow or Stonyfield Farms)
- No sugars, corn syrup, or artificial sweeteners, including agave nectar

FOODS YOU CAN EAT
- Proteins: Eat proteins according to your blood type: for instance, some meats are not so great for A blood types, but black beans are good. Use protein powders, but not with whey. Vegetable protein is great for A types. I love Life's Basics plant protein. If you don't know about blood types, read Eat Right for Your Type, by Dr. Peter L. D'Adamo. Fresh farm eggs (no hormones or antibiotics) are OK.

- FATS

Use coconut oil, extra-virgin olive oil, clarified butter, raw almonds (preferably soaked), and almond butter. Some people can handle raw peanut butter (not hydrogenated). Be careful with nuts because they're vulnerable to mold—add 1 tsp Silver Shield to every cup to kill any mold.

- BERRIES, LEMONS, LIMES, GRAPEFRUIT

These are very low in sugar and are the only fruits that are OK. Berries are great in smoothies with protein powder. Frozen berries are safer than fresh berries because fresh berries get moldy so easily. Limit fruits to 1 to 2 a day.

- VEGETABLES

Eat lots of veggies, especially the green leafy type because they promote oxygen. (Yeast thrives in an anaerobic/low oxygen environment). Don't eat starchy vegetables like potatoes, peas, and corn. Eat squash, sweet potatoes, and yams in small amounts—1/2 cup.

- OTHER

Add flavor and zip with real salt, pepper, Bragg amino acids, and herbs and spices. Rice milk, coconut milk, and feta cheese (goat, not cow) are OK. Eat small amounts of food every two to three hours. Approximately 80 percent of what you eat should be raw. Drink plenty of good water—distilled, or oxygenated, alkalized water if you can get it. Take high-quality supplements while doing the yeast cleanse, as they are an essential part of the process—Daily Supplements are recommended.

YEAST-FREE FOOD PLAN FOR THE LONG-HAUL

Removing harmful fungal yeast from your body is only half the battle. If you want it gone for good, you're going to have to change the way you eat forever. A long-term yeast-free eating plan (alkaline foods) might seem radical and unrealistic at first, but the human body was actually designed to eat this way, and once you get used to it, you'll be amazed at how good you feel.

Sugar, grains, dairy, and processed dead foods contain artificial flavors and preservatives that create acidic conditions that feed yeast. Eating a mostly bitter and alkaline diet will keep yeast at bay. To make it easy to figure out what you can and can't eat, just eat lots of dark green and bright orange vegetables and lean proteins, and steer away from sweets, breads, and processed foods. Typically, alkaline foods are alive (raw), and acidic foods are dead (cooked). But some acidic foods can be turned alkaline; for instance, beans, nuts, and grains become alkaline when they're soaked and sprouted.

Snacks are included in the yeast-free food plan because it's important to eat small amounts of nutritious food every 2–3 hours.

SAMPLE MENU (MAINTENANCE)

BREAKFAST
Eggs with veggies/feta (I like to add cilantro and salsa)
Oatmeal with berries or Granny Smith apples and cinnamon
Smoothies with Life's Basics protein powder, greens, and berries

LUNCH
Salad with veggies and protein, such as
hard boiled eggs or cooked dried beans
Lettuce wraps

DINNER
Meat and vegetables
Spaghetti squash with veggies and Italian red sauce
Grilled chicken with vegetables

SNACKS
Veggies with guacamole and salsa
Celery or carrots with hummus
Granny Smith apples
Raw nuts and seeds (preferably soaked)

ALKALINE FOODS
Lean protein
Good fats
Some fruits
Vegetables

CAN ALSO USE
Organic rice, coconut, and almond milk (unsweetened)
Goat-milk feta cheese
Good quality plain yogurt, like Brown
Cow, Stonyfield Farms, or Greek Yogurt
Vegan mayonnaise (Vegenaise)
Agave nectar, xylitol, and Stevia (don't overdo it)
Herbs and spices!
Bragg amino acids
Nut butters
Small amounts of whole grain breads, brown rice, and beans
(preferably sprouted)

*And we have made of ourselves living cesspools, and driven
doctors to invent names for our diseases.* Plato

HOW TO KEEP YEAST AWAY FOR GOOD

Health is not valued until sickness comes.
Dr. Thomas Fuller, 1654-1734

● USE NATURAL MEDICINES
Antibiotics, chemo, radiation, and many other medicines, including over-the-counter medicines, impair healthy cell function and disrupt balance in the digestive tract. Balance the body and support it in healing itself by practicing healthy habits and using herbs, essential oils, and energy work, etc. (Asterisks signify Nature's Sunshine products.)

● DO A CANDIDA CLEANSE
Take 5 drops lemon, 5 drops melaleuca, and 3 drops oregano in an empty gelatin capsule once a day for thirty days. Stop, and take probiotics for two weeks. Wait two weeks, and then repeat both cycles. Or just do a round of GI Cleansing Formula and Probiotic Defense Fomula instead of taking oils. Make sure you're eating yeast-free, exercising, and drinking plenty of pure water while on this cleanse. It won't work if the oils aren't high quality and pure.

● SUPPORT YOUR IMMUNE SYSTEM
An easy way to boost and improve your health is to add grapefruit and/or lemon to your drinking water. Also take these essential oils internally in a capsule (take 8-9 drops a day). L*Immune Stimulator contains beta glucans and is very important for immune support, especially if you have a weakened system.

● REPAIR LEAKY GUT
Probiotic Defense Formula and GI Cleansing Formula are designed to work together to clean and restore health to the

digestive tract—take GI Cleansing Formula for 10 days and then Probiotic Defense Formula for 5 days; then repeat at least once. Probiotics, astringent herbs, L-glutamine, and *Everybody's Fiber are also all very good for tissue repair (take on an empty stomach).

• IDENTIFY AND ELIMINATE FOOD ALLERGIES
After the cleanse, add foods back into your diet one at a time according to your blood type, and watch for yeast symptoms. If you pay attention, you will know immediately which foods work for you and which don't.

• SWITCH TO COLON-FRIENDLY SUGARS
Stevia, xylitol, agave nectar, and RAW honey are the most colon-friendly sugars. They are natural sugars that don't cause blood-sugar levels to spike or create unfavorable conditions in the colon when they're eaten in moderation. Eat all sweets, including fruits, sparingly.

• STAY AWAY FROM DAIRY
Avoid all dairy as much as possible, including whey. Dairy products create a gunky buildup in the digestive tract that yeast thrives on. Plain cultured yogurt or Keifer might be OK for you. Make sure you choose natural brands that are hormone and antibiotic free.

• AVOID PROCESSED AND REFINED FOODS
Processed foods, including canned foods, are mostly nutrient-void, and they create an acidic environment that's perfect for growing yeast.

• EXERCISE
Yeast thrives in a stagnant and lethargic atmosphere, so make sure you're really moving your body on a regular ba-

sis—at least 30 minutes, 3 times per week. Exercise helps the body to release toxins at a cellular level and creates an environment that's unappealing to yeast.

STRESS REDUCTION IS IMPORTANT!
- Make time for relaxation: try to rest for 20 minutes, 2 times per day.
- Get adequate sleep: aim for 7–8 hours a night.
- Take a sauna to raise body temperature: start slowly and build up—optimal is one hour per day, especially if you have a serious case.
- Have a positive attitude!
- Claim your power! Candida/parasites thrive in an emotional environment where a person feels unable or is unwilling to claim his or her power.
- Read Stress Free Living by Trevor Powell

Studies increasingly provide evidence that it is the additive and synergistic effects of the phytochemicals present in fruits and vegetables that are responsible for their potent antioxidant and anticancer activities. Our findings suggest that consumers may gain more significant health benefits by eating more fruits and vegetables and whole grain foods.
Dr. Rui Hai Liu, Cornell Associate Professor of Food Science

SUPER SUPPLEMENTS

Improve the medical system from a disease care system to a true health care system. Make the world a healthier and more peaceful place. Frank Lipman

Your body and brain require a proper balance of vitamins, minerals, enzymes, amino acids, and antioxidants in order for them to perform optimally. This means you need a diet rich in organic foods as well as well formulated and high-quality daily supplements.

When it comes to nutritional supplements, you don't always get what you pay for. In fact, testing done at independent labs has shown that the majority of supplements on the market, including very pricy supplements that are advertised as "the best of the best," don't contain everything that's listed on the label. This is because "fairy dusting" is very common in the industry. Fairy dusting is the practice of only putting in trace amounts of vitamins and minerals. In addition, many vitamin and mineral supplements contain cheap fillers and harmful chemicals.

There are long-term health problems associated with taking inferior quality supplements on a regular basis, which is why some professionals in the health field advise against taking nutritional supplements. Doctors and other health professionals are rightfully concerned about the dangers of taking poor quality supplements because taking them over an extended period of time can be harmful and actually contribute to disease rather than prevent it. This is why I highly recommend seeking out and supporting companies that are committed to quality and purity.

DAILY SUPPLEMENTS

The Daily Supplements I recommend are Cellular Vitality Complex, Essential Oil Omega Complex/Vegan Essential Oil Omega Complex, and Food Nutrient Complex.
My husband, Craig, and I have been taking these Daily Supplements for over 5 years now, and we would never consider giving them up! They have become must-haves at our house. They are so well formulated and pure (smart) that you don't have to be. All you have to do is take them regularly as recommended, and they get to work balancing and nourishing your body—and you start feeling and looking better.

CELLULAR VITALITY COMPLEX
Cellular Vitality Complex is an anti-inflammatory, antioxidant supplement. It contains potent levels of powerful polyphenols, or antioxidants that protect cells from free-radical damage. Free radicals are unstable molecules that damage cells and DNA and cause premature aging and disease, including chronic pain, heart disease, diabetes, autoimmune diseases, neurological diseases, and cancer. Cellular Vitality Complex helps prevent oxidation and inflammation caused by free radicals. It contains full therapeutic doses of the six most powerful polyphenols, namely resveratrol, quercetin, baicalin, epigallocatechin gallate (EGCG), ellagic acid, and curcumin.

ESSENTAIL OIL OMEGA COMPLEX
Essential Oil Omega Complex is a fish oil and Omega and Co-Q10 supplement. It contains a concentrated half-and-half blend of pure fish oils (EPA and DHA fatty acids) and marine oil (flaxseed oil, pomegranate seed oil, evening primrose oil, and cranberry seed oil) as well as a blend of clove, cumin, frankincense, German chamomile, ginger, thyme, and orange essen-

tial oils (these are antioxidant and anti-inflammatory oils that act as a protective natural preservative for essential fatty acids and enhance health when taken in a small daily dose). Essential Oil Omega Complex bioavailability is enhanced through a nanosomal lipid assimilation system encapsulated in vegetarian-friendly softgel that prevents fishy smell or aftertaste.

(FYI—Omega-3s are commonly found in olive oil, fish, and some nuts and seeds. Just so you know, even though fish is an excellent source of dietary omega-3 fatty acids, daily fish consumption as a source of omega-3 fatty acids is no longer advised because of the growing concern over the high levels of toxins and heavy metals in many of the world's oceans. In fact, many nutritional experts warn against frequent fish consumption because it risks exposure to toxic pollutants. If you're already taking fish oil, you should know that many fish oils on the market come from toxic and polluted sources. Essential Oil Omega Complex contains only clean and pure sources of concentrated fish oils.)

VEGAN ESSENTIAL OIL OMEGA COMPLEX

Vegan Essential Oil Omega Complex is a unique formula of therapeutic-grade essential oils and a proprietary blend of plant and algae-sourced omega fatty acids. Omega fatty acids help support healthy joint, cardiovascular, and brain health, support healthy immune function, and have been shown to help mediate a healthy inflammatory response in cells.

A single daily dose of Vegan Essential Oil Omega Complex provides 1200 milligrams of botanical omegas with 350 mg of ALA from flax seed oil and Incha Inchi oil, 20 mg of GLA from borage oil, 100 mg of DHA from algae, and a varied blend of other plant-sourced essential fatty acids. This complex also includes 800 IU of natural vitamin D, 60 IU of natural vitamin E, and 1 mg of pure astaxanthin, a powerful antioxidant carotenoid harvested from microalgae. The bioavailability of Vegan Essential Oil Omega Complex formula is enhanced through a nanosomal lipid assimilation system that is encapsulated in plant-based softgels.

FOOD NUTRIENT COMPLEX

Food Nutrient Complex is a vitamin and mineral supplement that contains a full therapeutic and optimally-balanced dose of vitamins and trace minerals, including chelated minerals and a tummy-taming blend of peppermint leaf, caraway seed, and ginger root extract—and no cheap fillers.

ESSENTIAL OIL CELLULAR COMPLEX

Essential Oil Cellular Complex is a proprietary blend of pure, therapeutic-grade essential oils that have been shown in clinical studies to help protect cells against free radical damage while supporting healthy cellular function. The blend includes clove, thyme, and orange essential oil with limonene, which provides powerful antioxidants that help protect cellular DNA from free-radical damage. It also includes essential oils from Boswellia serrata (Indian frankincense), lemongrass, summer savory, and niaouli, which have been shown to support cellular apoptosis and renewal.

Essential Oil Cellular Complex is an important supplement because you can only be as healthy as your cells are!

Essential Oil Cellular Complex essential oil blend is useful for rubbing along the spine or on the bottoms of the feet and over afflicted areas. It also comes in a liquid capsule form that includes a nanosomal lipid assimilation (delivery) system for improved bioavailability and digestion and is handy to take along with other supplements every day. One 8-drop serving (480 mg) of Essential Oil Cellular Complex has a very impressive ORAC 5.0 score of over 5,000!

Just so you know, if I had cancer, you can bet that no matter what, taking generous doses of Essential Oil Cellular Complex, along with frankincense and Daily Supplements, would be at the top of my list!

ENERGY & STAMINA COMPLEX

Energy & Stamina Complex provides a safe and natural way to increase low energy. It has a nourishing effect on cells and is completely different than caffeine and amphetamines, which are commonly taken to burst energy levels but are detrimental to health.

Unlike caffeine, which stresses the nervous system, Energy & Stamina Complex increases mental acuity. Following is a list of the primary benefits:

• Promotes efficient production of ATP (perfect energy production) in the mitochondria (energy factories) of cells
• Enhances stamina and the efficient use of oxygen in cells
• Supports metabolic adaptation for diverse activities; it is helpful with everything from movie watching to marathon running
• Adaptive—helps the body adjust to stressors
• Enhances immunity
• Reduces cortisol levels—promotes calmness
• Reduces/balances blood sugar
• Increases memory and mental clarity
• Enhances receptor activity
• Antioxidant
• Aphrodisiac

What makes Energy & Stamina Complex unique is that it contains high levels of acetyl-L-carnitine, cordyceps, American ginseng root extract, ginkgo leaf extract, ashwagandha root extract, alpha-lipoic acid, coenzyme Q10, and quercetin dihydrate in a proprietary blend. Acetyl-L-carnitine is a primary ingredient that supports mitochondrial function by helping transport fat into the mitochondria to burn for energy. Energy & Stamina Complex contains ashwagandha root extract, which has been called the "herb of the ages" due to its ability to boost energy levels and support immunity and libido, as well as reduce anxiety, insomnia, and stress. Perhaps its biggest benefit however is its ability to support the regeneration of cells from damage caused by free radicals. This is important for people dealing with cancer. Energy & Stamina Complex comes in sodium lauryl sulfate–free vegetable capsules and does not contain ingredients made from milk, wheat, or animal products.

PROBIOTIC DEFENSE FORMULA & GI CLEANSING FORMULA
Probiotic Defense Formula and GI Cleansing Formula are designed to work together to help support a healthy digestive tract. This, in turn, strengthens the body and helps prevent/counteract superbugs. For best results, take a round of GI Cleansing Formula for ten days and then a round of Probiotic Defense Formula for five days. It is suggested that you wait for at least ten days before repeating rounds.

PROBIOTIC DEFENSE FORMULA
Probiotic Defense Formula contains five proprietary strains of friendly probiotic microorganisms that support healthy digestive function and immunities. Probiotic Defense Formula comes in a patented, time-release beadlet that's shown to be safe and beneficial to people of all ages.

The primary benefits of Probiotic Defense Formula are that it supports healthy digestive functions and immunities while creating an unfavorable environment for unhealthy bacteria, yeast, and other harmful microorganisms. It also helps boost GI immunities to prevent digestive infections such as traveler's diarrhea and helps manage the unpleasant symptoms of irritable bowel syndrome.

Probiotic Defense Formula helps support optimal absorption of food nutrients and energy metabolism and helps support healthy skin conditions (many skin issues stem from an overgrowth of Candida yeast).

GI CLEANSING FORMULA

GI Cleansing Formula is a blend of therapeutic-grade essential oils and caprylic acid that help support a healthy digestive tract by creating an unfriendly environment for potentially harmful pathogens. GI Cleansing Formula contains a proprietary blend of therapeutic-grade essential oils from oregano, melaleuca, lemon, lemongrass, peppermint, and thyme. Each of these oils has been shown to improve microbial balance. Caprylic acid is a naturally derived fatty acid from coconut oil that's known to positively affect digestive health. It has antimicrobial activity and has been used for over 40 years to improve microbial balance of the digestive tract. GI Cleansing Formula is a proprietary blend that helps to purify and cleanse the digestive system.

FYI—Probiotics (acidophilus, bifidophilus, etc.) build good bacteria in the gut, which in turn fights off bad bacteria, including Candida yeast. Probiotics strengthen the immune system so that the body can fight off superbugs. Superbugs prey on people with weak immune systems (toxic guts); but people who have healthy colons and strong immune systems can host superbugs without any problem. In fact, people with strong immune systems are so immune to superbugs that the bacteria can actually live on their skin and in their noses without them being infected!

Think about your immune system like this: At all times you have a war going on in your digestive tract, with Candida yeast being the bad guys and probiotics being the good guys. If you have a ratio of 90 percent probiotics and 10 percent Candida, you will never get sick. If you have a ratio of 80 percent probiotics and 20 percent Candida, you will still most likely be well most of the time. But if your ratio is 60 percent probiotics and 40 percent Candida, you'll be prone to "catch" everything that comes along.

In our day and age, a ratio of 90 percent probiotics and 10 percent Candida is not very realistic for most people. A ratio of 80 percent probiotics and 20 percent Candida is realistic, but it requires actively taking steps to achieve and maintain it. The best way to achieve and maintain a healthy balance of bacteria in your colon is to avoid prescription antibiotics, sugar, and junk foods and to take a good probiotic with each meal. If you are taking measures to build a healthy immune system, you will be far less likely to get sick.

DIGESTIVE ENZYME COMPLEX

Digestive Enzyme Complex is a proprietary blend of eight active whole-food enzymes that are often deficient in cooked, processed, and preservative-laden foods. Digestive Enzyme Complex includes a variety of whole-food enzymes that support healthy digestion and the metabolism of enzyme-deficient, processed foods, which in turn helps with the digestion of proteins, fats, complex carbohydrates, sugars, fiber, and other food nutrients.

Digestive Enzyme Complex contains a patented enzyme assimilation system of whole-food minerals that are necessary cofactors for enzymatic activity throughout the body. It promotes gastrointestinal comfort and food tolerance and is a powerful combination of eight active whole-food enzymes and a blend of peppermint, ginger, and caraway seed extracts that promote gastrointestinal comfort.

Digestive Enzyme Complex is safe for all members of the family, including babies, and generally doesn't interfere with medications. Digestive Enzyme Complex is a whole-food formula made with sodium lauryl sulfate–free HPMC vegetable capsules and can be used as targeted support for specific food intolerances of proteins, fats, and carbohydrates such as lactose. Digestive enzymes should be taken right before meals. You don't have to worry about taking too many because it's very hard to overdo it. In addition to helping with digestion, enzymes are important aids for strengthening the immune system.

Ideally, digestive enzymes should be taken before every meal, and they should be stored in a cool, dry area to ensure potency.

Digestive Enzyme Complex contains the following enzymes, which are listed along with the activity they support:

• Protease – breaks down protein into peptides and amino acids
• Amylase – breaks down carbohydrates, starches, and sugars
• Lipase – breaks down fats and oils to be absorbed in the intestine
• Lactase – breaks down lactose found in milk sugars
• Alpha Galactosidase – breaks down complex polysaccharide sugars found in legumes and cruciferous vegetables that can cause bloating and gas
• Cellulase – breaks down fiber to help digest fruits and vegetables
• Maltase – breaks down maltose sugars into glucose for energy
• Sucrase – breaks down sucrose to fructose and glucose for energy

FYI—Enzymes are essential to life, and they play a role in practically all body functions. The body manufactures its own supply of enzymes, however, because enzymes are the only nutrients that can supply the body with energy. Overuse can impair their functioning capacity, which can lead to numerous disorders and diseases.

Heat above 119 degrees destroys most enzymes, which is why cooked foods, including anything that's been homogenized or pasteurized, cannot be relied on as sources of enzymes. Raw plant foods such as green leafy vegetables are optimal sources of enzymes, and the more raw leafy green foods you eat, the more enzymes you will get. And the more enzymes you get, the healthier you'll be!

DETOXIFICATION COMPLEX

Detoxification Complex (SLS-free capsule) is a proprietary blend of whole-food extracts in a patented enzyme delivery system that supports healthy cleansing and filtering functions of the liver, kidneys, colon, lungs, and skin.

Here's why Detoxification Complex is an important supplement: The human body has a filtering system (immune system) that's job is to get rid of harmful toxins and germs. Problems occur, however, when immunity becomes weakened and can't properly perform its function. In addition, the filtering organs get clogged and dirty, much like a filter on your furnace or car. Detoxification Complex and Detoxification Blend support the immune system and cleanse and support the body's filtering organs.

Following is a list of each targeted organ, along with herbs or whole-food extracts that support it. Each was selected specifically to provide protective cleansing and filtering of the body's functions and to support the organ's own capacity to rid itself of stored toxic waste products.

- Liver – barberry leaf, milk thistle seed, burdock root, clove bud, dandelion root, garlic fruit, red clover leaf
- Kidneys – Turkish rhubarb stem, burdock root, clove bud, dandelion root
- Colon – psyllium seed husk, Turkish rhubarb stem, acacia gum bark, marshmallow root
- Lungs – osha root, safflower petals
- Skin – kelp, milk thistle seed, burdock root, clove bud, garlic fruit

DETOXIFICATION ESSENTIAL OIL BLEND
Detoxification Blend is a proprietary blend of therapeutic-grade essential oils of clove, grapefruit, rosemary, and geranium that have been studied for their support of the cleansing organs of the body. This blend is formulated to be used individually or in combination with Detoxification Complex. The recommended dosage is 5 drops of Detoxification Blend taken in the evening in an empty capsule.

FYI—Detoxification Complex is formulated to be used in conjunction with Detoxification Blend; however, individual products can be used separately. For optimal benefits, eat organic plant foods and avoid processed foods that contain artificial colors, preservatives, and sweeteners. Also avoid chemicals in cleaners and hygiene products, and drink plenty of pure water.

COLLOIDAL SILVER
Silver, in its colloidal form, has been proven useful against many different infections. It has been shown that disease-causing bacteria cannot live in the presence of even minute traces of metallic silver. Silver is nontoxic in reasonable concentrations against all species of fungi, bacteria, protozoa, parasites, and certain viruses. The concentration of

twenty parts of silver per million contained is a highly-effective and safe formulation. Higher concentrations are actually less effective because they can interfere with beneficial bacteria and cause skin to turn blue.

Our culture has gone way too far in its war on germs. The end result is bacterial imbalances that are implicated in everything from allergies and asthma to chronic fatigue and heart disease. [The book] The Probiotics Revolution is must reading for everyone who is interested in achieving or maintaining vibrant health. Christiane Northrup, MD, Women's Bodies, Women's Wisdom, and The Wisdom of Menopause

Probiotics represent the next wave of health and healing. Whether you are concerned about your immune system, digestion, hormones, allergies, or skin, [the book] The Probiotics Revolution provides cutting-edge research with down home and practical solutions. Ann Louise Gittleman, PhD, CNS, The Fat Flush Plan

KITCHEN HERBS THAT FIGHT CANCER

The following kitchen herbs and spices taste great, and studies in university laboratories show that they have anticancer properties as well.

- **OREGANO**
Scientific studies have repeatedly shown that oregano is possibly the most potent anticancer herb. Oregano contains many powerful antioxidant vitamins and is effective in the prevention of cancer, as well as in slowing down the aging process. Studies show that ounce for ounce oregano is one of the most antioxidant-rich foods; one tablespoon of oregano was found to have as many cancer-fighting antioxidants as an apple. Oregano also has strong antibacterial properties that inhibit the growth of bacteria, including those that cause food-borne illness.

Oregano goes especially well with tomato-based sauces, which enables you to easily add cancer-fighting properties to everything from pasta to salsa. Use all parts of the oregano plant—fresh herbs are most potent. Oregano and other leafy herbs, including mint, thyme, marjoram, and basil, contain terpenes, a substance that works on tumors by encouraging cancer cells to kill themselves.

Pure oregano essential oil provides an easy way to use this powerful cancer- and infection-fighting herb in a concentrated form. Oregano essential oil can be taken internally in a capsule and can also be applied topically (such as on the bottoms of the feet); but it is an extremely hot oil, so make sure you never put it over a rash or open wound. Oregano can be "cut" or diluted with a carrier oil.

The human body is the best picture of the human soul.
Ludwig Wittgenstein

• ROSEMARY

Rosemary is an antispasmodic, "tonic" herb with powerful antioxidant properties. Studies have proven that rosemary fights bacteria and cancerous tumor growth and significantly reduces breast cancer development. Research has also revealed that marinating uncooked meat in rosemary significantly reduces cancer-causing compounds.

Rosemary acts as an astringent and decongestant. It helps prevent liver toxicity and is good for headaches, high and low blood pressure, circulatory problems, and menstrual cramps. It relaxes the stomach and stimulates circulation and digestion. It also relieves menstrual cramps, tired nerves, impaired nerve function, nerve or muscle tension or pain, fevers, the flu, and headaches. Rosemary improves circulation to the brain and is a good brain or memory tonic.

Rosemary is good on vegetables and in pasta sauces. Rosemary essential oil inhibits skin tumors and protects DNA against strand breaks (prevents cancer). It induces detoxification enzymes and is calming and relaxing. Pure rosemary essential oil can be taken internally in capsules.

• GINGER

Studies done at the University of Michigan Comprehensive Cancer Center and the University of Minnesota's Hormel Institute showed that ginger has anticancer properties and is effective for treating a variety of cancers. It was noted that the compound gingerol, which gives ginger its distinct flavor, has an anticancer effect on colorectal, breast, prostate, and ovarian cancers.

Ginger can be added to stir-fry dishes, healthy soups, fresh juices, and green smoothies. Ginger essential oil is a highly diverse essential oil that's good for relieving topical pain, motion sickness, nausea, upset stomach, and flatulence. Pure ginger essential oil can be taken topically in a capsule.

- GARLIC

Garlic is antiviral, antibacterial, antifungal, and expectorant. It has been shown to fight precancerous cells and to prevent cancer-causing compounds from forming in the body. Garlic, onions, leeks, shallots, and chives belong to the allium family. Alliums contain quercetin and allicin, which are strong antioxidants and anti-inflammatory agents that prevent the formation of carcinogens and that cause cancer cells to die. Garlic fights infection by detoxifying the body and enhancing its immune function. No drug can match garlic's power to protect the body against heart disease and strokes. Garlic reduces cholesterol, prevents blood clots, controls diabetes, and helps prevent cancer. Garlic is, in fact, good for virtually any disease or infection!

When onions and garlic are cooked and eaten with other foods, they help lower insulin peaks and prevent uncontrolled cell growth and inflammation, which would make a person vulnerable to cancer. Garlic is a versatile seasoning that goes well with almost all kinds of foods—from Italian to Chinese. For the most benefits, eat garlic raw; cooking can reduce its potent anticancer activity. Powdered garlic can be taken in a capsule.

- TURMERIC

Turmeric contains curcumin, a compound that has a strong preventative effect on colon, breast, lung, stomach, skin, and prostate cancers. Studies show that a teaspoon of turmeric per day can prevent the development of some cancers.

Turmeric is a major flavoring in Indian curries. It can be taken like an herb, in a capsule.

Optimum health begins with a good foundation. Andrew Weil, MD

- CHILI PEPPERS—JALAPENOS

Capsaicin, which is the chemical that makes hot peppers so spicy, has been shown to neutralize certain cancer-causing substances called nitrosamines and also to help prevent cancers such as stomach, pancreatic, skin, and ovarian cancers. Hot peppers literally cause cancer cells to self-heal, while being perfectly safe for normal cells.

Cayenne is a great cleansing and strengthening tonic herb that comes from hot peppers and has different degrees of heat. If you take too much of a hot type of cayenne, it can be very caustic. If you do overdo it with a hot pepper, drink water and organic unprocessed apple cider vinegar (neutralizes and stops spasms), and take musilous herbs such as phyllium hulls, slippery elm, marshmallow, fenugreek, and aloe vera. Musilous herbs absorb irritants and toxins and relieve inflammation, so they're good to have on-hand.

Chili peppers are good in cuisines ranging from Mexican to Asian. Ground up chili peppers can be taken in capsules—just don't overdo it with a very hot type.

- CINNAMON

Cinnamon contains phenolic polymers, which are beneficial for type 2 diabetes and cardiovascular diseases. Cinnamon can reduce blood sugar and LDL cholesterol levels, as well as increase insulin levels. Proanthocyanidins, a type of flavonoids in cinnamon, have a potent antioxidant capability and may be able to inhibit tumor growth by starving cancer cells. These special flavonoids may also block the formation of nitrosamines, which is a carcinogen that can damage the DNA in breast tissue.

Cinnamon can be used in stick or powdered form, both of which are derived from cinnamon bark. It is delicious in a wide variety of baked goods and marinades.

MEDICINAL HERBS THAT FIGHT CANCER

Essiac (tea) is an excellent blood cleanser and can help tremendously if someone is toxic from either chemotherapy or radiation. Patients seem to feel better taking Essiac; at some level it appears to enhance mood. Dr Jesse Stoff, MD

- ESSIAC

Essiac® is an herbal blend discovered by Rene Caisse, a Canadian nurse (essiac is caisse spelt backwards). Essiac is primarily made up of burdock root, slippery elm, sheep sorrel, and Indian rhubarb root. In a Cancer Clinic in Canada, Rene used Essiac to successfully treat thousands of patients suffering from cancer. The following is excerpted from an article she wrote, which was published at the time of her death in 1979.

> "From 1934 to 1942 I paid the Council the sum of $1.00 per month for the building and there was a large "CANCER CLINIC" sign on the door. I treated thousands of patients who came from far and near, most of them given up as hopeless after everything in medical science had failed. Some arrived in ambulances, receiving their first treatments lying down in an ambulance; after a few treatments they walked into the clinic without help.
>
> I had absolute faith that I could accumulate enough proof of results obtained with different types of cancer, as demanded by the Cancer Society, the medical profession would eventually be glad to accept Essiac as an approved treatment.

I did not know then of an organized effort to keep a cancer cure from being discovered, especially by an independent researcher not affiliated with any organization supported by private of public funds. Tremendous sums have been raised and appropriated for official cancer research during the past 50 years, with almost nothing new or productive discovered. It would make these foundations look pretty silly, if an obscure Canadian nurse discovered an effective treatment for cancer!" (See www.essiacinfo.org/caisse.html)

• ALFALFA

The renowned herbalist Dr. John Christopher considered alfalfa to be the king of herbs. It is loaded with vitamins and minerals, including vitamins A, B-1, B-6, C, E and K, calcium, potassium, iron, zinc, and amino acids. Alfalfa is also a good source of chlorophyll, fiber and protein. It is a powerful blood and liver cleanser that neutralizes acids and poisons and carries waste out of the body and helps restore healthy pH. Thus it is an important herbal supplement for treating cancer and maintaining overall good health.

• BARLEY JUICE POWDER

Barley grass is the seedling of the barley plant. It is a concentrated source of vitamins and minerals and is particularly rich in vitamins A, C, B1, B2, folic acid, B12, calcium, iron, potassium, chlorophyll, and all nine essential amino acids (which the body can't produce). Barley grass is a powerful antioxidant that can help the body kill cancer cells and regain health and vitality

My opinion is that [herbs] are superior 95 percent of the time to any pharmaceutical drug! Dr. Willner, MD

• BURDOCK

Burdock (root) is a powerful blood and liver cleanser that quickly eliminates toxins from the body. It contains an abundant supply of nutrients, including biotin, copper, essential oils, inulin, iron, manganese, sulfur, tannins, zinc, and vitamins B1, B6, B12, and E. Burdock balances hormones and is good for glandular problems. Burdock poultices are very effective for skin cancers.

• CHAPARRAL

Chaparral is a deep blood cleanser and detoxifier that attacks free radicals and stimulates the production of healthy cells. Several university studies have shown that chaparral has the ability to dissolve cancerous tumors. Interestingly, the FDA has been working to get chaparral taken off the market.

• GARLIC

Garlic is an antiviral, antibiotic herb that strengthens white blood cells and protects the body against cancer. Traditionally, garlic was used for the treatment of cancer. In fact, Hippocrates, who is widely referred to as the Father of Modern Medicine, used garlic to treat cancerous tumors. Many consider garlic to be one of the most healing foods in the world.

• KELP

Kelp is a seaweed that has the ability to dissolve poisons and toxins in the body (it's a powerful blood cleanser). Kelp is a very nourishing herb that promotes healthy thyroid function as well as healthy hair, skin, and nails. It protects against stress and environmental toxins and promotes an overall balanced and healthy system.

Much virtue in herbs, little in man. Benjamin Franklin

● PAU D' ARCO

Pau D' Arco is a blood purifier and blood builder that protects the liver. It has successfully been used in hospitals in South America to treat cancer victims. When it's taken along with chemotherapy, Pau D' Arco seems to stop the damage done by chemotherapy. It also appears that Pau D' Arco reduces tumors by dissolving them.

● RED CLOVER

Red clover is a powerful blood cleanser that's widely known to be effective for treating all types of cancer. It's been shown to be especially beneficial when combined with chaparral and dong quai. Red clover is a highly-nutritious plant that's good for all degenerative diseases. It's also a great nerve tonic.

● SUMA

Suma is an ancient herb that purifies and strengthens the entire body. It is an "adaptogen" herb, which means it relieves stress and energizes and normalizes all of the systems in the body. Suma is known to inhibit cancer cell growth and to be effective for many types of cancers.

Chaparral has been used for centuries without incident by Native American Indians as well as by millions of cancer victims. In fact, it is estimated that over 200 tons (500 million capsules) have been sold in the U.S. in the last two decades alone. Dr. Norman Farnsworth¹s extensive studies on chaparral in the 1970s and 1980s were unable to find any hepatotoxic properties. Dr Rona, MD

ESSENTIAL OILS

Essential oils are the oldest medicine known to man. They are useful for virtually every condition and known to safely kill germs, viruses, and infections, including funguses, while building the immune system.

Modern scientists who have been investigating the incredible healing powers of essential oils enthusiastically endorse them and their amazing benefits! For instance, did you know that clinical research has shown that frankincense contains very high immune-stimulating properties, and viruses cannot live in the presence of cinnamon oil?

Another thing that's very impressive about essential oils is how fast they work. When they are applied to the skin, they immediately penetrate into the body and travel through the blood stream; and within about twenty minutes, they have positively affected every cell in the body!

Essential oils are easy to use, and they're good medicine for everything. There are three primary ways to use essential oils:

TOPICALLY
You can rub essential oils on the bottoms of the feet, along the spine, on the fleshy part of the ears, and over painful or afflicted areas. You can also add them to bathwater (mix with a little Epsom salt first) and wear them as perfume to raise your body's vibrational level and increase your immunity.

AROMATICALLY
You can diffuse essential oils to elevate your mood and clean the air, because essential oils safely remove harmful bacteria, mold spores, offensive odors, metallic particles, and toxins, and they increase beneficial oxygen and ozone and positively affect the amygdala gland like nothing else can.

INTERNALLY

Many brands warn against internal consumption, but therapeutic-grade essential oils actually have FDA approved nutritional labels on them. Truly pure essential oils can safely be taken internally (in a capsule, etc.) to relieve internal pain and further penetrate healing of deep organ cells.

FYI—The reason most essential oils warn against internal consumption is because they contain synthetics and can be very harmful to the body. On the other hand, 100% pure, truly high quality essential oils are perfectly safe to take internally as medicine.

Another thing I love about essential oils is that they are very cost effective. One 250-drop (15 ml) bottle can be used for multiple conditions, and it generally costs less than a co-pay for a doctors visit or prescription. Even more expensive oils don't seem so costly when you compare them to medicine and consider all the miraculous things they can do.

Drugs never cure disease. They merely hush the voice of nature's protest, and pull down the danger signals she erects along the pathway of transgression.
Any poison taken into the system has to be reckoned with later on even though it palliates present symptoms. Pain may disappear, but the patient is left in a worse condition, though unconscious of it at the time. Daniel. H. Kress, MD

ESSENTIAL OILS ARE NOT ALL THE SAME

In order to be labeled "pure, therapeutic-grade," all essential oils must pass a gas chromatograph test. This is the industry standard. Unfortunately, the gas chromatograph test is such a basic test that synthetic and chemically distilled oils can easily pass it. This explains why the majority of essential oils labeled "pure, therapeutic-grade" really aren't pure or high-end at all. It's a fact that most essential oils on the market have gone through a cheap chemical-distillation process that's rendered them synthetic and low-grade.

Synthetic oils might smell like the real thing to an untrained nose, but they can actually be harmful, rather than helpful, to the body. You can generally tell poor quality essential oils by their oily (sticky), rancid (old and stale smelling), bitter tasting, and perfumey nature.

While the gas chromatograph test is an incomprehensive and incomplete test, the mass spectrometry test picks up on every impurity and also shows the exact amount of every constituent in an essential oil. The mass spectrometry test is expensive and not required, so most companies don't even consider it. I have found that the best essential oils have passed both the gas chromatograph and mass spectrometry tests with flying colors. Truly pure, therapeutic-grade essential oils contain nutrition labels on the bottle that say they are safe to take internally as medicine. Less pure (synthetic) brands actually warn against internal consumption.

In case you're wondering which oils are best, go online and read what other people are saying about quality. Keep in mind that when A LOT of people are singing a company's praises… and the main rhetoric is coming from their competition, it's a pretty good indicator that the company and their oils/wellness products are really good!

ABOUT FREQUENCIES

Dr. Royal R. Rife was a scientist who invented the Universal Microscope in 1993. Dr. Rife's research showed that every disease and substance has a frequency and that substances with higher frequencies destroy diseases of a lower frequency. In his book, The Body Electric, Dr. Robert O. Becker explains that the human body has an electrical frequency and that a person's level of health can be determined by that frequency.

In 1992, Bruce Tainio of Tainio Technology, an independent division of Eastern State University in Cheny, Washington, built the first frequency monitor in the world. Through his studies, Tainio determined that a healthy body's frequency is in the range of 62–72 Hz. And the frequency of the average human body during the daytime is 62–68 Hz. He realized that when the body's frequency drops, the immune system becomes compromised.

When the frequency drops to 58 Hz, cold and flu symptoms start to appear; at 55 Hz, diseases like Candida take hold; at 52 Hz, autoimmune diseases and herpes occur; and at 42 Hz, the body gets very serious diseases like cancer, HIV, and AIDS.

Knowing about frequencies helps us realize that the quality of the air we breathe, the food we eat, the water we drink, and everything we are exposed to, in general, matters. For instance, processed/canned foods have a frequency of zero, while fresh produce (greens) has a frequency of up to 15 Hz. Dry herbs measure from 12 to 22 Hz, while fresh herbs range from 20 to 27 Hz. Obviously, foods with the highest frequencies are the healthiest.

Clinical research has shown that pure essential oils have the highest frequency of any natural substance known to man. Pure essential oils start at 52 Hz. and go to as high as 320 Hz. High quality rose oil is 320 Hz; it has the highest frequency of any substance on the planet. Not only do pure essential oils provide the fastest way to raise frequencies, oxygenate cells, and improve immune health, but they also create an environment in which disease, bacteria, viruses, and fungi, cannot survive. Essential oils are 50–70 times more concentrated than herbs, and using them on a daily basis is one of the easiest ways to raise your body's vibrational level! The numbers listed below are frequencies. They will help you see just how much your frequency affects your health.

FREQUENCIES IN THE BODY

The numbers listed below are frequencies and will help you see just how much your frequency affects your health. As you can see, low frequencies, acidity, and weakened immune systems are synonymous with poor health.

If you are experiencing health problems and would like to become healthier, you must alkalize your system and raise your body's frequency. This requires a lifestyle change. While you're at it, make sure you help your kids upgrade their lifestyle too. Home is the best place for them to learn good habits, and they will benefit as much as you do!

62–72 = Strong and healthy body
• Strong and healthy immune system

58 = Susceptible to colds and flu
• Weakened immune system
Candida Cleanse recommended

55 = Candida yeast is present
• Critically weakened immune system
Candida Cleanse needed

52 = Autoimmune diseases develop
• Impaired immune system
Candida Cleanse needed

42 = Cancer and AIDS develop
• Critically impaired immune system
Cancer Protocol needed!

The highest form of ignorance is to reject something you know nothing about. Wayne Dyer

HOW TO RAISE YOUR FREQUENCY & BOOST YOUR IMMUNE SYSTEM

The average frequency of the human body during the daytime is between 62 and 68 cycles each second. If it drops below this rate, the immune defense system will start to shut down. Cold symptoms appear at 58 cycles, flu at 57, Candida at 55, glandular fever at 52, cancer at 42 cycles each second. Bruce Tainio

Simply taking well-balanced nutritional supplements and using pure essential oils on a daily basis will help rid your body of toxins and also raise your frequency and strengthen your immune system. High quality nutritional supplements and pure, therapeutic-grade essential oils are good preventative medicine.

● AVOID JUNK FOOD
Processed foods, sugary junk foods, soda, energy drinks, coffee, and alcohol are all very acidic, and they GREATLY contribute to lowered body frequencies and weakened immune systems—if you want to get healthier, you must stop eating/drinking them. As much as possible, eat a yeast-free diet, and

don't microwave your food. Drink water instead of juices and soda pop.

- DO THE CANDIDA CLEANSE
People who have been diagnosed with cancer, diabetes, lupus, arthritis, rheumatoid arthritis, headaches, Crohn's disease, colitis, fibromyalgia, and many other autoimmune diseases have noticed dramatic improvements after switching to a yeast-free diet and doing the Candida cleanse.

- EAT A YEAST-FREE DIET
A yeast-free food plan might seem radical and unrealistic at first, but most people who try it are surprised at how good they feel and at how easy it is to "eat clean."

- TAKE SUPPLEMENTS; USE PURE ESSENTIAL OILS
Simply taking well-balanced supplements and using pure essential oils on a daily basis will help rid your body of toxins, and also raise your frequency and strengthen your immune system. High quality nutritional supplements and essential oils are also very good preventative medicine.

- ADJUST YOUR ATTITUDE; ADOPT HEALTHIER HABITS
Don't stress. Chill, and find healthy ways to release negative emotions. Take time to laugh and play. Listen to wholesome music and motivational speeches. Aim to be positive, happy, and generous always; give as good as you hope to get. Get up and move around! Make sure you're getting plenty of pure water, sleep, exercise, fresh air, and sunshine. Help others who need a helping hand, and spend time with people you love. Keep growing and reaching upwards; take classes, read from good books, and expand your mind. Meditate and pray.

In minds crammed with thoughts, organs clogged with toxins, and bodies stiffened with neglect, there is just no space for anything else.
Alison Rose Levy, An Ancient Cure for Modern Life

CANCER MEDICINE, ESSENTIAL OIL STYLE

My own prescription for health is less paperwork and more running barefoot through the grass. Leslie Grimutter

It is common knowledge that chemotherapy kills healthy cells along with the cancerous cells. It is not unusual for cancer therapies to kill a large percentage of good cells along with the bad, which is why hair loss, yellow eyes, grayed hair, nausea, fatigue, and other symptoms are typical among patients of chemotherapy. It is exciting news that some essential oils have been shown to kill cancer cells without harming healthy cells!

A team of scientists from the University of Oklahoma Health Sciences Center and the Oklahoma City VA Medical Center, headed by Dr. HK Lin, evaluated frankincense oil's impact on both normal human bladder cells and cancerous human bladder cells in culture. The results showed that frankincense essential oil was harmless to the normal cells, but it zeroed in on and killed the cancer cells.

Dr. Jaime Matta, Ponce School of Medicine, Ponce, Puerto Rico, also found frankincense very effective for killing cancer, even chemotherapy-resistant strains of breast cancer.

Not only have essential oils been shown to be a successful treatment for cancer, but when therapeutic-grade essential oils are used to treat cancer, the cell death count is less than 25 cells! And according to the research done by Nicole Stevens, MS, even when essential oils are repeatedly used at extremely high concentrations, there are no toxicity levels! In addition to frankincense, sandalwood, thyme, lavender, and clove are also antitumor oils. Rosemary and clove have been shown to prevent cancer, and frankincense and lavender encourage the rapid regrowth of healthy cells.

Frankincense and sandalwood are both expensive oils, because the process of properly distilling them is very time and labor intensive. Research has shown that other less-expensive oils such as marjoram, thyme, lavender, clove, orange, and peppermint can be combined with frankincense and sandalwood and can actually increase their effectiveness as a cancer treatment!

When essential oils are combined with Daily Supplements and a healthy diet and lifestyle, they form a very powerful and effective formula for healing!

As scientists and doctors are experiencing the miraculous benefits of essential oils, they are publishing them in medical journals, and it is having a positive effect on the way the medical community is viewing the healing power of essential oils. If you are interested in more information about essential oils and cancer research, please go to www.aromaticscience.com.

He is the best physician who knows the worthlessness of his own medicine. Professor W. M. Osler, Professor of Medicine, Oxford University

FRANKINCENSE ESSENTIAL OIL

Frankincense oil may represent an inexpensive alternative therapy for patients currently suffering from bladder cancer. Dr. HK Lin

Throughout the ages, frankincense has been used as a sacred religious offering; and to this day, frankincense is still considered a most precious gift, fit for a king or for God. The Bible mentions frankincense as a "gift" brought by wise men that traveled from the east to worship baby Jesus. Frankincense has long been used as a sacred religious offering. To this day, frankincense is still considered a most precious gift, fit for a king—or for God.

The wise men who worshiped baby Jesus very likely traveled from Oman, Jordan. Oman is a desert region in the east known to produce the best frankincense in the world. Records show that frankincense has been harvested in Oman since as far back as 7,000 BC.

Harvesting frankincense is a skill and livelihood that's been passed down through generations of families living in Dhofar, Oman. The reason why frankincense is so expensive is that it's very time and labor intensive to harvest it.

Oman's frankincense is a very versatile oil that promotes rapid tissue growth. It can be applied topically as well as taken internally in a capsule. Taking frankincense internally nourishes and heals deep organ cells, particularly those associated with the throat, kidney, liver, and digestive and urogenital tracts.

Given all of the scientific research done on this powerful oil, if I had cancer, I would take about 5 drops (or more) of pure, therapeutic-grade frankincense (from Oman... with a nutritional label on the bottle) in a capsule, two to three times a day.

Wellness Made Simple

I'd also apply it directly over the cancerous area. At the very least, I would take PURE, therapeutic-grade frankincense internally every day if I had cancer!

Cancer starts when the DNA code within the cell's nucleus becomes corrupted. It seems frankincense has a re-set function. It can tell the cell what the right DNA code should be. Frankincense separates the 'brain' of the cancerous cell (the nucleus), from the 'body' (the cytoplasm), and closes down the nucleus to stop it reproducing corrupted DNA codes.
Mahmoud Suhail, immunologist

CANCER PROTOCOL

When 100% pure essential oils are combined with a healthy diet and lifestyle and good nutritional supplementation, you have a very powerful and effective formula for healing!

That said, the following cancer protocol has been used to successfully rid some people's bodies of cancer. If you want to try the cancer protocol, I strongly suggest combining it with the following:

• The yeast-free diet (no sugar or junk food!)
• Essential oil spinal technique (do it daily)
• High quality nutritional supplements, including non-synthetic vitamins and minerals, e-omegas, and antioxidant-rich cellular support (take daily)
• Pure water—drink 3/4 of body weight in ounces of distilled water or filtered water that's similar to Kangen 9.5 water, daily (pulls toxins)

The entire protocol can be repeated as often as necessary. It is strongly advisable that you only use 100% pure, therapeutic-grade essential oils that have been approved for internal consumption, because this will not work if you use inferior oils. Plus, inferior oils could cause more sickness.

• Day 1–3: Take one 00 capsule with frankincense, one 00 capsule with sandalwood, and one 00 capsule with lavender—do this morning and evening for 3 days. Also apply frankincense, sandalwood, and lavender topically, morning and evening, over cancerous area, during the 3 days

• Day 4–6: Repeat the same process as days 1–3, using frankincense and sandalwood, but replacing lavender with orange

• Day 7–9: Repeat the above process, using frankincense and sandalwood, but replacing orange with lemon

• Day 10–12: Repeat the above process, using frankincense and sandalwood, but replacing lemon with thyme

• Day 13–16: Repeat the above process, using frankincense and sandalwood, but replacing thyme with clove

At the end of 16 days, follow up with a package of Probiotic Defense Formula, which is a powerful probiotic that will further heal and strengthen the body

FOR PAIN—some combinations of oils may work better than others. Experiment with the following blends and adjust amounts if you need to. The trick is to find what works best for whoever is suffering. Try as needed:

- Do the Aroma Massage treatment for pain

- Apply topically 8 drops of white fir and 4 drops of frankincense

- Take internally in a capsule 12 drops of wintergreen, 8 drops of vetiver, and 8 drops of helichrysum

- For nerve-type pain, take 6 drops of vetiver, 6 drops of peppermint, and 6 drops of Soothing Blend in a capsule; also apply these oils topically

FYI—I did some research and found out the only reason wintergreen and birch have childproof caps is because companies that sell natural products containing large amounts of methyl salicylate are "by law" required to label them "for external use only." This is all because of an FDA ruling, which was the result of a runner massively overusing and overdosing on synthetic pain-relief rubs.

An autopsy done on the runner showed that there was a toxic amount of methyl salicylate in her system. Ironically, the FDA didn't rule against the synthetic rubs she'd been using, just methyl salicylate in a natural form.

After a group of doctors got together and appealed the ruling, arguing that wintergreen and birch are much safer than over-the-counter pain relievers, which are known to cause harmful side effects, yet have been given the stamp of approval by the FDA, the FDA rescinded the ruling. Still, by law, companies that sell wintergreen oil have to label it for external use only.

That said, wintergreen has strong cortisone-like properties, and it is an excellent pain reliever. I have personally taken a capsule full at a time internally, and it's worked amazingly well with no harmful side effects. Based on my own experience, I believe it is perfectly safe to take (100% pure) wintergreen internally.

"CANCER PROTOCOL" TESTIMONIAL

This testimonial was taken with permission from an email support group:

"For those of you who have blessed me with a major amount of info, I wanted to send an update on my pa, Joe. He was doing so good for the past three months, but now he has started to decline quickly. He was on the protocol for 3 months and continues to have an Aroma Massage treatment every day, sometimes 2 times a day (for pain). He also has white fir and frankincense rubbed softly on his legs and back (where the cancer is the worst); this has helped with pain in a major way. He has had to up his morphine as well, to ward off the worst of the inside pain. The morphine is barely touching his pain at this time.

His protein counts have all gone up this month, and his X-rays now show that the cancer has invaded his spine as well as his shoulders, legs and other areas. He is preparing not to be with us for much longer at this time.

Now for those that asked was it worth doing the cancer protocol, YES! I think that 3 months of being able to enjoy life to the fullest, go on a trip with my ma, and to be able to work and paint was worth any amount of money. Do I think the protocol worked, yes, to the extent that it could for my pa. When we started the protocol he was in the hospital with possibly days to live, he had a problem with his lungs, a weak heart, and infection in his blood! He was sent home with no other options and was not given any hope to live. He went on the protocol in his last stages of the cancer, and it made his life good for three great months.

I want to encourage those that are thinking of this cancer protocol to start it at the diagnosis stage. Don't wait until the cancer invades all the areas of your body. Although this is not a medical claim by any means, it is an encouragement to take charge of your health. I still believe that this protocol when used at the diagnosis stage makes a huge difference, just think what the outcome might have been if I had known of this protocol years ago when my pa was diagnosed with his bone cancer.

The cancer protocol helped my ma have 3 awesome more months with my pa. As the cancer is now in his spine and shoulders, I will now just ask for prayer for his pain. Thank you again for the amazing portal of information you all are!"

DAILY REGIME FOR CELLULAR HEALTH

Everyone can benefit from practicing a daily regime for health, because 80 percent of health problems can be avoided just by practicing preventative measures!

A cleansing and healing regime is important because it restores health to an unhealthy body. As a rule of thumb, after an initial three-month cleansing period, it will take one month for every year that you've had problems for your body to heal.

The following daily essential oil and supplement regime is a cost- and time-effective way to prevent and heal disease. It will help you create health at the cellular level. It will also enable you gain control of your money and your family's health!

Here is the daily regime:

DAILY SUPPLEMENTS
This is a vitally important part of a wellness regime! Take Daily Supplements as directed

• Supplies body with antioxidants
• Stimulates proper metabolic function

- Contains natural fatty acids
- Everyday vitamins & minerals
- Heart health
- Digestive aid
- Anti-inflammatory
- Boosts energy
- Addresses chronic pain

CITRUS OILS
Take 10–15 drops a day in water (or a capsule)—use lemon, lime, bergamot, orange, or grapefruit

- Natural cleanser and detoxifier
- Aids in eliminating heavy metals
- Stress reduction

GROUNDING BLEND
Apply 2–3 drops to the bottoms of the feet

- Grounding
- Antidepressant
- Regulates hormones
- Repairs wear and tear on central nervous system

CALMING BLEND
Apply 1–2 drops nightly to the bottoms of the feet; use lavender, rosemary, patchouli, or Focus Blend OR make your own relaxing blend

- Aids with sleeplessness
- Antidepressant

Relaxing Blend Recipe
15 drops Roman chamomile
20 drops bergamot
25 drops frankincense
Mix blend in a roller bottle—can be diluted with coconut oil

PROTECTIVE BLEND
Apply 2–3 drops along the spine and then on the bottoms of the feet

- Stabilizes the immune system
- Diffuse to eliminate germs

FRANKINCENSE
Take 2–3 drops under the tongue twice a day, or apply to the neck at the base of the skull

- Decreases anxiety
- Improves circulation
- Reduces chronic inflammation
- Reduces joint pain

ESSENTIAL OIL CELLULAR COMPLEX
Take as directed 2 times a day, morning and night

- Protects and repairs cells

DETOXIFICATION COMPLEX
Take 1 capsule two times a day for 20 days. Repeat a round of Detoxification Complex quarterly

- Supports and cleanses toxins from filtering organs of the body: liver, kidney, bladder, blood, and colon

DETOXIFICATION BLEND
Take 5 drops daily in a capsule with dinner

• Supports healthy cleansing and filtering functions of the liver, kidney, bladder, blood, and colon

DIGESTIVE ENZYME COMPLEX
Take 1–3 capsules before every meal

• Supports healthy digestion of food nutrients
• Aids in conversion of nutrients into energy

GI CLEANSING FORMULA & PROBIOTIC DEFENSE FORMULA
Repeat a round of GI Cleansing Formula and Probiotic Defense Formula monthly

• Heals the intestinal tract, which is important for reversing all diseases.

GI CLEANSING FORMULA
Take 1–3 capsules 3 times a day with meals, for 10 days

• Clears Candida yeast
• Cleanses intestinal tract (If it makes you feel sick, don't worry—It means its working!)

PROBIOTIC DEFENSE FORMULA
Take 2 times a day for 5 days

• Restores probiotics to the intestinal tract

CORIANDER
Apply 1–2 drops on the bottoms of the feet 2 times a week. If you have diabetes or any other blood sugar issue, use coriander daily—you can take it in a capsule

• Regulates blood sugar (take with Metabolic Blend)
• Aids in eliminating heavy metals

Happiness lies, first of all, in health. George William Curtis
ESSENTIAL OILS FOR EMOTIONAL WELLNESS

TO REDUCE FATIGUE
Try peppermint, lemon, or Invigorating Blend

TO REDUCE STRESS
Try Joyful Blend, ylang ylang, Massage Blend, Tension Blend, or basil

TO INCREASE PEACE
Try Calming Blend, Roman chamomile, Joyful Blend, orange, frankincense, or Grounding Blend

TO INCREASE PASSION
Try ginger, basil, Invigorating Blend, peppermint, or Joyful Blend

TO INCREASE DOPAMINE LEVELS (PLEASURE)
Try rosemary, Roman chamomile, clary sage, or patchouli

TO INCREASE SERATONIN LEVELS (RELAX)
Try lavender, orange, marjoram, Roman chamomile, or thyme

TO INCREASE NOREPINEPHRINE LEVELS (ENERGY)
Try lemongrass or rosemary

ZERO-POINT ENERGY

Zero-point energy is a unique form of energy that exists only in the vacuum of empty space. It is the energy of nothingness and can be embedded into devices—such as wands, pendulums, and nutritional products—to relieve pain and to heal disease in the body. When the body is exposed to zero-point energy, or when zero-point energy is ingested, this ideal energy transfers to the cells and causes the electrical charge across cell membranes to remain at an optimal level, which then enables cells to release toxins and to fully absorb nutrients—thus every cell in the body experiences significantly increased health and vitality.

Studies have shown that "energy work" using zero-point energy products can actually change a person's genetic structure. Because the effects of energy healing can be measured, more and more experts in the field of hard science are paying attention to zero-point energy and acknowledging its validity.

The zero-point energy products I am familiar with is the Amega AMized™ wand. The Amega wand looks and feels a lot like an ordinary silver pen, but it's made up of a mixture of granulated minerals encased in stainless steel.

The wand has been shown to emit 1250 mega hertz of energy (frequency) and to increase immunity and have a calming effect on the nervous system. When the wand is used on the body or on any living organism, it acts as a memory switch that invites cells to remember where they came from. This, quite simply, unblocks meridians and creates homeostasis, which is a balanced and high-frequency state that enables the body to self-heal.

To use the wand, you simply point it towards the area where you are experiencing pain (hold it close), and then rotate it in a clockwise motion from 3 to 18 times. It literally only takes minutes for the pain to go away, and oftentimes for good!

You can also clear blocked energy in the body's meridians and energy fields by pressing the tip of the wand into the tips of each finger and toe (one at a time), rotating it clockwise at least 3 times and then flicking it off.

The wand is more effective when used in conjunction with essential oils—together they have a powerful synergetic effect. It's also beneficial to wand your food, drinking water, bathwater (it can get wet), plants, pets, and chakras—just point toward an object, or each chakra, and circle about twelve times.

When I first saw the wand, I thought it looked hokey, but I could feel it doing something to me, and I liked the concept; so I bought one to use on my clients during massages. I was surprised when they all reported they could feel I was doing something different to them when I hadn't even told them. One client said each time I pointed it, it felt like I was dropping essential oils on her back.

SELF-HELP OXYGEN THERAPY FOR CELLS

The FDA won't spend a dime on ozone research, but they spent over $1 million intimidating, harassing, and persecuting me alone. Dr. Jonathen Wright

The bloodstream carries nutrients necessary to utilize oxygen to the body's cells. Oxygenated blood is clean and healthy and flows easily, whereas un-oxygenated blood is low in nutrients, toxic, and sluggish. If you have sluggish and toxic blood, you probably don't feel so good. If you want to feel better, you must clean up your blood (cleanse) and then change your habits so that your blood will stay clean and oxygenated.

One of the best ways to oxygenate the blood is through regular cardiovascular exercise! Getting your heart rate up and keeping it up for an extended period of time naturally cleanses and oxygenates blood. Other ways of oxygenating the blood include taking liquid oxygen, getting oxygen treatments, and using pure essential oils and zero-point energy products (just apply oils and wand yourself regularly to quickly oxygenate blood cells).

In all living, have much fun and laughter. Life is to be enjoyed, not just endured. Gordon B. Hinckley

OXYGENATE WITH ASEA

You can change your state in so many ways,
and they're all so simple. If you've been consistently focusing
on the worst that could happen, there's no excuse for continu-
ing to do that. Start now to focus on the best.
Tony Robbins

ASEA is a liquid supplement that oxygenates/heals blood and raises the body's frequency. It slows down aging and increases health by reducing oxidative stress and regenerating cells after cellular damage. Research has shown that ASEA increases the effectiveness of the body's natural antioxidants by over 500 percent. This is a big deal because antioxidants produced by the body (like glutathione, SOD and catalase) are far more powerful than antioxidants introduced from outside sources. Thus, ASEA is being touted as an unparalleled immune-boosting product.

I became sold on ASEA after seeing several life-slides of blood before and after people had taken ASEA. Within minutes after taking the product just one time, the difference in their blood was profound! I also saw blood samples of people who had been on the product for about three months, and in each case there were masses of dead parasites. Obviously, ASEA cleans up and heals blood. This is important because clean, healthy blood is foundational.

The woman who showed me the slides said she had been doing live-blood analysis for several years, and during that time she's observed that when people take herbs it takes months for their blood to change; but with energy-work, the change is immediate. She said emotions and music are especially powerful—that when people think peaceful or loving thoughts or listens to harmonious music such as classical and hymns, their blood begins to repair itself. But when people feel upset or angry or listens to inharmonious music, especially acid rock, it immediately causes their blood to deteriorate and start breaking down.

Here's how the blood and ASEA work: There is an unceasing traffic of molecules and ions that travel in and out of each cell through its plasma membrane. All cells acquire the molecules and ions they need from their surrounding extracellular fluid. Through this process, the membrane connects to cells and downloads DNA and then turns into whatever it's coded or "programmed" to become, which is how disease or wellness is created within us.

ASEA is a stabilized sodium chloride solution. Sodium chloride supplies the body with electrolytes. When sodium chloride is stabilized, it changes the electrical charges in the body through an ion-binding process. This causes redux signaling, which literally changes DNA coding and prevents even hereditary diseases from happening. In short, ASEA changes the communication between cells, which greatly affects and improves the blood, demonstraring a significant healing effect on a person's overall health!

The woman showing the blood slides said that in her years of testing she's never seen a substance that affects the blood like ASEA does; she said that after people take ASEA, their white blood cells become supercharged, and there is an immediate improvement in their red blood cells. She pointed out that you can actually see the cells communicating and restructuring (and it certainly looked like that's what they were doing).

The best way to absorb ASEA is to take an ounce, a mouthful at a time, and swish it around in your mouth (including under your tongue) for about a minute before swallowing it. I've found that it's usually best to take doses at least an hour apart and to finish with the last dose by about 2:30 p.m. The pH Miracle, by Robert Young and Shelly Young, will help you understand ASEA's full effect on blood.

THE POWER OF EXERCISE

With the new day comes new strength and new thoughts.
Eleanor Roosevelt

Regular exercise benefits every part of the body. It oxygenates the blood. It prevents and improves chronic health conditions. It strengthens the hearts and lungs and increases energy. It helps prevent and manage high blood pressure and cholesterol. Regular exercise boosts high-density lipoprotein (HDL or good cholesterol) while decreasing low-density lipoprotein (LDL or bad cholesterol). It lowers the buildup of plaques in the arteries and helps prevent type 2 diabetes as well as osteoporosis and certain types of cancer. Exercise also reduces feelings of depression and anxiety, and it can really improve bad or depressed moods. Regular exercise burns calories and helps keep weight under control. It makes us look and feel better, and it boosts our confidence and self-esteem. Being fit even makes sex more enjoyable.

Regardless of your age, gender, or physical ability, you can do some form of exercise. Whether you do an intense class or workout at the gym or you jog or take a walk or go for a hike or do a DVD at home or park far away or take the stairs instead of the elevator, you are moving your body and burning calories—and it's all good! For optimal results, you should exercise at least 30 minutes a day, five days a week, and alternate between weight training, aerobic exercises (including walking), and yoga or stretching. At the very least, get up and stretch and move around (try doing jumping jacks, squats, and lunges) several times throughout the day.

Exercise doesn't have to be hard work; in fact, it can actually be lots of fun. If you find it difficult to get motivated, sign up for a class or find an exercise partner and set up regular times to workout. If you have special needs, Google "exercise programs for people with special needs."

BENEFITS OF WEIGHT LIFTING (weight machines, dumbbells, or resistance bands)
• Increases strength and fitness • Improves muscular endurance • Increases bone density • Improves posture • Improves balance and coordination • Shapes and tones muscles • Burns fat • Increases energy levels • Gets results fast • Decreases pain • Reverses and slows down aging • Reduces risk of diseases like heart disease, diabetes, and cancer • Reverses problems caused by diseases

BENEFITS OF CARDIO/AEROBICS (30–60 minute sessions)
• Raises metabolic rate—burns a lot of calories • Burns fat fast • Decreases risk of cardiovascular disease • Increases balance and coordination • Improves posture • Makes the body sweat, cleansing the skin and making it glow • Decreases depression • Releases feel-good endorphins • Reverses and slows down aging • Increases self-confidence • Increases self-esteem

BENEFITS OF YOGA/PILATES (stretching and toning)
• Tones muscles • Increases flexibility • Increases strength • Lubricates joints, tendons, and ligaments • Strengthens core muscles • Improves posture • Improves balance • Massages all organs of the body • Detoxifies all parts of the body • Reverses and slows down aging • Harmonizes body, mind, and spirit

If you want to get the best out of a man,
you must look for the best that is in him. Bernard Haldane

THE POWER OF MEDITATION

Excessive talk and hurry are enemies of wisdom. Philip McCoy

Meditation is the practice of quieting the mind. It is the art of shutting off chatter and sitting quietly by yourself. It is moving into a space of simply being. Essential oils can help enhance the experience. Good choices are Invigorating Blend (on the heart center) and Grounding Blend (on the bottoms of feet). If you have frankincense, it's also useful to put a drop of oil on the center of the forehead and/or on the top of the head. Using essential oils will create higher states of peace and consciousness during meditation.

• LET GO
You can completely relax and sit in silence and think about nothing at all. Try becoming centered by quietly listening to soft music—music that mimics nature is always nice.

• IMAGINE
Guided imagery is a technique that involves using mental images to promote deep relaxation. Guided imagery effectively uses the power of the mind to release physical pain and to begin self-healing in the body. It creates changes in attitudes or behaviors and can be facilitated by a guided visualization CD or trained therapist.

The following guided imagery meditation doesn't require assistance and is ideal to do in the morning or evening or whenever you're feeling upset. Simply close your eyes and take a few deep conscious breaths. Notice where there's pain or tension in your body, and let it go. Envision all sad, fearful, judgmental, guilty, or other inharmonious energy flowing out of you. In your mind, picture Jesus Christ standing in front of you and taking all the inharmonious energy away. Envision Him replacing it with love and light. Picture a thick cord of light running through you, connecting you to heaven, earth, and to all the goodness and wisdom the universe has to offer. Envision heavenly angels surrounding you, anxiously waiting to help and protect you. Feel their love, and silently thank them for continually serving you.

Offer a silent prayer of gratitude for the blessing of being alive. Ask God to be with you and to help you make the most of your day. Breathe in light and love, and picture it swirling all around you. Feel it filling your entire body. Relish in the feeling of being alive. When you are ready to face the world again, open your eyes and notice all the wonderful things God is sending your way. Remember to continue on with an attitude of gratitude!

● BREATHE

Mindful breathing is another form of meditation that's very beneficial. To begin, try setting a timer and spending five minutes doing nothing but thinking about your breath. Keep your eyes and mouth closed, and breathe in deeply through your nose and hold it; then breathe out through your nose and hold—in and hold, and out and hold, then in and hold, and so forth. If five minutes is too long, try breathing for at least one or two minutes, and then gradually build up to more.

It's through the breath that we let go of stress and receive peace. If you don't believe me, try angrily clenching your jaw and keeping it that way while you're slowly and deeply B-R-E-A-T-H-I-N-G in and out. You'll find it's pretty hard to do, because as you deeply breathe in, peace automatically flows in; and as you slowly breathe out, tension automatically leaves your body with your breath. As you take a big breath in, picture bright clean light flowing into your body through the top of your head and down into your stomach. As you hold, feel clean air filling your chest cavity and nourishing your heart. As you slowly breathe out, feel your stomach emptying, and picture your burdens and all the painful energy you've been holding on to release out through your feet. Picture all heavy and negative energy flowing into the earth to be cleansed and repolarized. As you B-R-E-A-T-H-E in and out, imagine things you'd like to experience and picture them flowing toward you. If you want better health, picture your body in a strong and healthy state. Imagine the universe (or your body) reorganizing to accommodate your positive desires. Trust that your wants are important; and with God's help, you can create and attract an abundance of good and rewarding experiences, including good health. Breathe, and be at peace.

What I've learned this year is that my weight issue isn't about eating less or working out harder, or even about a malfunctioning thyroid. It's about my life being out of balance, with too much work and not enough play, not enough time to calm down. I let the well run dry. Oprah Winfrey

THE POWER OF HEARTFELT PRAYER

Prayer does not use up artificial energy, doesn't burn up any fossil fuel, doesn't pollute. Neither does song, neither does love, neither does the dance. Margaret Mead

Over the past decade, hundreds of scientific studies have been performed at some of the nation's top universities, and they have repeatedly shown that prayer is powerful and effective medicine. Prayer changes things. Time after time it has been shown that people who are prayed for heal at a much faster rate than those who are not prayed for.

In addition, many studies have shown that people who pray regularly tend to be happier and more satisfied with life. Studies also suggest that people who pray and attend religious services on a regular basis are healthier and live longer than those who don't, regardless of their age, health, habits, or demographics.

Prayer is simple and powerful, and it's free medicine. If you aren't in the habit of praying, now is the perfect time to start. As far as praying goes, there's no exact wording or right formula for personal prayers; the main thing is that they need to come from your heart.

Gratitude and respect are key elements to effective prayer. As long as you are respectfully talking to your Heavenly Father from your heart, it's impossible to do it wrong. It is human nature to question God and wonder why He would allow bad things to happen, and it is fine to respectfully pray out upsets or concerns, including feelings of anger, frustration, confusion, and sadness. It is never okay to curse or mock God through prayers or otherwise, though. And being bitter and disrespectful won't get you the positive results you're looking for.

THE POWER OF LOVE!

Love never dies a natural death. It dies because we don't know how to replenish its source. It dies of blindness and errors and betrayals. It dies of illness and wounds; it dies of weariness, of witherings, of tarnishings. Anais Nin

In The Hidden Messages in Water, Dr. Emoto uses photographs to illustrate how lovely white crystals form whenever molecules of water are exposed to the words love and gratitude—which are the highest vibrational words. Obviously the energy of love is HARMONIOUS, GRACEFUL, DELIGHT-

FUL, and EASY. It's no wonder that love makes us feel so warm and fuzzy inside!

To love and be loved feels terrific—with good reason. Being in love actually lowers our stress hormones, decreases our blood pressure, increases our energy, and spurs on our desire to be physically active. Love also makes us feel less depressed and less inclined to participate in destructive behaviors such as smoking and drinking.

Given this fact, it's not surprising that research has shown that when we catch the "love bug," our happiness increases and so does our immune health!

The nice thing about love is that the more we exercise our "love muscles," or, in other words, the more we feel and express genuine love toward others (and forgive them of their imperfections), the more love and good health we get in return. Yes, indeed, love makes the world go round, and giving and receiving love makes being alive a joyful and extremely worthwhile experience!

When it comes to loving, it is impossible to truly love others if you don't wholeheartedly love yourself. In fact, it is the exact amount of love and respect you have for yourself that radiates out and determines how much love and respect you feel for God and for everyone else.

When it comes to self-love, I often think of these now-famous words, penned by Marianne Williamson: "We ask ourselves, who am I to be brilliant, gorgeous, talented and fabulous? Actually, who are we not to be? You are a child of God. Your playing small doesn't serve the world . . . We were born to make manifest the Glory of God that is within us . . . And as we let our light shine, we unconsciously give people permission to do the same." (A Return to Love)

If you are suffering from a lack of love in your life, there's no better time than now for you to start falling in love with yourself! If you don't truly value, cherish, and respect yourself and wholeheartedly think you are someone really great, you can't truly "shine" (be radiantly happy) or pass love and light and inspiration on. And no matter how much someone else loves you, you won't be able to fully receive, feel, or enjoy it.

In case you are in the habit of criticizing or downplaying yourself, or negatively projecting the future, determine to stop right now. Turn over a new leaf and start a love journal for the sole purpose of helping you fall in love with you! Start by making a list of every good trait or quality you see in yourself.

As you mindfully look for good things, you'll notice more and more of them. Write them all down. Also write down the good qualities you'd like to possess. Ask yourself what you would do if you knew you could not fail? Keep in mind that the happiest people are not those who have a lot of "stuff" but rather those who are reaching out and making the world a better place.

When you are serving others just for the sake of giving, you'll find that it's easy to feel happy and loving towards yourself. And when you are happy and in love with yourself, you'll find that you want to reach out and give more (love) again and again; and, consequently, you'll receive all the love and appreciation you need to be radiantly healthy!

THE POWER OF FORGIVENESS

When you hold resentment toward another, you are
bound to that person or condition by an emotional link that
is stronger than steel. Forgiveness is the only way to dissolve
that link and get free. Catherine Ponder

It's easy to be offended and hurt by the cruel or thoughtless acts of others. It's also easy for most of us (even those of us with the best of intentions) to occasionally act in a thoughtless and insensitive manner that inflicts pain on someone else.

Making mistakes, being hurt, hurting others, and then feeling negative emotions such as anger, resentment, bitterness, and/or guilty remorse is a natural and normal part of life. It's just part of the human experience.

Thank goodness for forgiveness, which is a high-frequency heart-action that soothes wounds and makes pain and negative emotions go away.

Forgiveness is not excusing, forgetting, or pretending that an offense never occurred—nor is it blindly trusting someone after they have abused you. Forgiveness is simply giving up the desire to get revenge and hurt others after they have done something hurtful. It is the act of surrendering hostile and negative feelings and replacing them with acceptance and love.

If you want to heal or remain healthy, you must learn to repeatedly forgive others (and yourself) for not being perfect. Forgiveness isn't necessarily easy, but it is always possible—especially when you sincerely pray and ask God for help. True forgiveness is absolutely necessary if you want to achieve and maintain overall good health.

To forgive is the highest, most beautiful form of love. In return,
you will receive untold peace and happiness. Robert Muller

THE POWER OF LIGHT

The sun has been demonized for years and as a result, people have avoided any direct exposure to sunlight. I think that's the wrong message. Michael F. Holick, Boston University School of Medicine

Cancer patients need LIGHT! According to a scientific article in Health & Diet Times, written by Lee de Vries, MD (June/July 1982), cancer cells self-destruct within minutes after exposure to strong intense light.

The sun is the brightest light in the universe, and unprotected exposure to strong sunlight, in moderation, is super good for you—and the majority of sunblocks aren't. While it's true that excessive tanning and overexposure to the sun can cause skin damage and certain types of skin cancer, it's also a fact that some regular unprotected exposure to the sun is known to prevent skin cancer and premature aging, and most sunblocks actually do more harm than good!

We've been brainwashed to believe that the sun will kill us and that sunblocks are good for us; but the truth is that sunblocks block beneficial UBA rays that help our bodies produce vitamin D, which is absolutely essential for good immune health as well as for the prevention of aging and skin cancer! And sunblocks contain toxic chemicals that readily absorb through the skin and build up in the bodies' organs—and consequently cause premature aging and disease. Many experts agree that a little unprotected daily sun exposure is the best and most effective way to get enough vitamin D. Coincidentally, exposure to natural sunlight has also been shown to increase calcium absorption.

Research has shown that poor diets, lethargic lifestyles, negative attitudes, trashed immune systems, and Candida yeast (over-acidity) are behind cancers of all types. And as far as wrinkles and skin damage goes, yes, repeated overexposure to the sun does cause wrinkles and such—and so does dehydration, poor diet, sugar, lack of sleep, toxic overload, ill-temperedness, and stress. So if you're concerned about your health and beauty, keep in mind that OVER-exposure to the sun, sunburns, sunblocks and chemicals, poor eating, and negative thinking are known to cause skin cancer and early wrinkles. And healthy eating, positive thinking, exercise, clean living habits, and moderate unprotected sun exposure are known to prevent it—and they cause "radiance" that cosmetics and sunblock cannot buy!

Rather than slather on thick layers of sunblock every time you go outside, make sure you're eating right, exercising, sleeping, drinking enough pure water, and being positive and happy. (Brush your teeth and smile—that alone is a great beautifier and health-enhancer!) Starting in the early spring, make it a point to get out in the sun for 15–20 minutes a day so you can build up to a base tan. (I'm just talking about getting a little color here and not a deep dark tan.) If you get used to being in the sun in the spring when it's less intense, as it gets hotter and brighter it won't bother you; and you'll be able to absorb its healing benefits without having to worry about burning. Even people with sensitive skin can build up a resistance to the sun this way.

I am not saying that you should never use sunblock. In fact, when you're going to be in the sun for an extended period of time, especially if you're fair skinned or don't have a base tan, you definitely should protect yourself. But it's important that you don't overdo it, especially with sunblock that contains harmful chemicals.

When choosing a sunblock, keep in mind that over 90 percent of commercial sunblocks contain octyl methoxycinnamate (OMC), which is a chemical that keeps the body from manufacturing its own essential Vitamin D. And even in low doses, OMC has been shown to kill mouse cells, especially when mice are exposed to sunshine! Commercial sunblocks also typically contain butyl methoxydibenzoylmethane, which is a toxic "filter" that is absorbed through the skin and circulates through the bloodstream. They also contain dioxybensone and oxybenzone, which are known to be extremely potent free-radicals, or destroyers of health. Before you buy sunblock, it's always a good idea to read the label. Mineral-based sunblocks and sunscreens made with ingredients you are familiar with and can pronounce are the safest.

Regarding the sun, I have a very good little book that, unfortunately, was out of print the last time I checked. It is titled The Body Is the Barometer of the Soul, and it was written by an Australian author, Annette Noontil. Regarding the sun, Annette makes an interesting assumption that I agree with.

"The sun has changed and the radiation from the sun is different. Sun cancers are a result of your inability to adapt to the changing conditions. The new sun is for new age thinking, different from the old age. Those people who embrace the new thinking will have little or no problem with their skin. Those who resist that change will have change thrust upon them."

Annette's point of view makes sense. We are "children of the LIGHT." Think about it. As a whole, we tend to get down and depressed during gray and gloomy winter months when sunlight is dim, but *we come to life when the sun gets bright and the weather warms up!*

Our world literally revolves around the light of the sun! It is impossible for us to live or grow (thrive) without it, and we certainly can't get away from it. So why would God make us so extremely incompatible with it?

In addition to getting plenty of bright sunlight, it is advisable to get enough healthy fats, particularly flaxseed oil, coQ10, and Omega 3s. If you can't get out in the sun during the winter, or if you live in a non-sunny climate, you might want to try lying on a light table occasionally. Light tables and even tanning beds provide good ways to absorb bright light. You might also need to take extra vitamin D.

As far as the sun, vitamin D, and cancer connection go, Dr. John Cannel has posted a very interesting video on YouTube. To watch it go to www.youtube.com and type "Dr. John Cannel on vitamin D" in the search box.

Get as much exposure to sunlight and fresh air as you possibly can and watch your tumors and cancers shrink away. Dr. Jürgen Buche

THE POWER OF POSITIVE THINKING

Stress is not caused by events, but by your response to events. Anonymous

When it comes to your overall health and happiness, your attitude is a very important factor. If you are a "worrier," you should know that the word worrying comes from an old English word that means to "kill by strangulation," which is fitting because it's just what constant chronic worrying does.

Worrying exhausts and paralyzes us to the point that it twists us up, wrings us dry, and prevents us from enjoying life and using our God-given abilities to solve our problems. Ironically, most of the things we worry about never come to pass because they're only in our minds. Or they do happen simply because we create them by constantly worrying and thinking about them? And, as for fear, it is an extremely low vibrational emotion that's just False Evidence Appearing Real! Worrying and fearfulness creates negativity, "checked-outness," unhappiness, and depression.

Unhappiness, checked-outness, and depression are conditions that plague our society and are often treated as a disease. The accepted treatment is to prescribe drugs that further numb and depress the mind and spirit. But a pill doesn't fix the problem, because it can't erase negativity and checked-outness and switch on optimism, vitality, and happiness.

If you're one who gets so down that you can't just smile and pull up joy, take heart because even a desire and determination to be happy can help you overcome unsettling feelings of fear and hopelessness. Counting your blessings and keeping a gratitude journal rather than wallowing in your pain really helps when you're feeling down. Getting dressed up and leaving your house and doing something to bring someone else joy is also very helpful. Exercise, proper nutrition, and being surrounded by positive and upbeat people and influences are essential. And, of course, sincere prayer is a powerful tool that brings peace, comfort, hope, and improved attitude like nothing else can.

It's a fact that people who choose to be positive, outgoing, and happy are typically content with their circumstances. And negative, discontent, and unhappy people aren't—no matter how good their circumstances are. Happy people don't necessarily have it better than unhappy people do, they're just better at seeing the bright side and blooming where they're planted. And their ability to be optimistic and adaptable no matter what happens nets them better health and more rewarding experiences and relationships—and an increase in things to be happy about. No wonder when Harvard introduced its first class on happiness in 2006 it quickly became Harvard's most popular subject. Obviously, most people want to be happy.

If you suffer from unhappiness and depression and would like to feel lighter and more joyful, you'll need to forgo self-apathy and "fixes" and start revamping your attitude and lifestyle.

Make sure that you're supporting yourself by eating right, taking good supplements, cleansing when you need to, constantly exposing yourself to positive people, and getting plenty of exercise, sleep, and pure water—as all of these things will help you overcome disinterest in life.

Happiness is a feeling that starts from within and begins with you choosing to feel pumped-up and good. If you repeatedly choose to get UP and take care of yourself, and notice and feel gratitude for your blessings, it is inevitable that you'll begin to feel a higher level of joy within—and thus create a more enjoyable and rewarding future for yourself. You are not a victim to down-heartedness; you can always choose to look up and do what it takes to feel happy!

If you have been diagnosed with cancer or any other disease, do not "own" the cancer or let it become your identity. Instead refer to it as "the" cancer and not "my" cancer. Words and thoughts are powerful forms of vibrations that have can shape the future, so it's in your best interest to choose your words wisely. Make it a point to only label yourself positively, with words and thoughts that express the way you'd optimally like to feel and be.

As soon as you start to feel differently about what you already have, you will start to attract more of the good things, more of the things you can be grateful for. Joe Vitale

Wellness Made Simple

THE POWER OF LAUGHTER

Laughter in and of itself cannot cure cancer nor prevent cancer, but laughter as part of the full range of positive emotions including hope, love, faith, strong will to live, determination and purpose, can be a significant and indispensable aspect of the total fight for recovery. Harold H. Benjamin, PhD

Hearing the words "you have cancer" is possibly one of the un-funniest things that can happen to a person. However, several studies have shown that the ability to laugh in spite of it has healing power, and a positive attitude can greatly boost your chances of overcoming it. In one study, among patients with rapidly spreading cancers, the people who expressed the most hope at the time of their diagnosis survived the longest.

Dr. Bernie Siegel, author of Faith, Hope & Healing, emphasizes the importance of hope, determination, optimism and a "fighting spirit" among patients battling cancer. People who deal with cancer by being optimistic and positive are the most likely to be long-term survivors with no relapses. On the other hand, people who submit to the news that they have cancer with an attitude of helplessness and hopelessness are more likely to die quickly or to have cancer come back with a vengeance after remission.

Life happens, and we all get to experience both good and bad things. How we choose to deal with the ups and downs of life either makes us better or bitter. Choosing to see the humor in a difficult situation eases the pain. And choosing to make lemonade out of lemons can turn a sour experience into one that tastes sweet.

When you let go and wholeheartedly laugh, you experience the emotion of JOY. Coincidentally, studies have shown that feeling high levels of joy automatically releases an increased amount of natural cancer-killing cells into the bloodstream!

More than one person has used laughter to heal cancer. Remember the lady in the movie The Secret who giggled herself well while watching comedies? Not only does laughter boost the immune system, but it also can't help but release tension and stress.

In a study done on patients in a rehabilitation hospital, 74 percent agreed that sometimes laughing works as well as a pain pill. These patients were suffering from a broad range of conditions—such as spinal cord injury, traumatic brain injury, arthritis, limb amputations, and other neurological or musculo-skeletal disorders.

There is a story told of a Methodist minister who was in a serious accident and had to spend several weeks in the hospital. He was in a lot of pain and was given pain shots to reduce it. The procedure was always the same. When the pain got bad enough, he would ring a buzzer near his bed, and a nurse would soon come to give him the shot. One day, he rang for the nurse and then rolled over on his side (with his back to the door), pulled his hospital gown up over his exposed backside, and waited for the nurse to come in. When he heard the door open, he pointed to his right bare buttock and said, "Why don't you give me the shot right here this time?"

After a few moments of silence, he looked up. It was a woman from his church! Following a brief embarrassing conversation, the woman left, and the minister, realizing what he had done, started laughing. He laughed so hard that tears were coming out of his eyes when the nurse arrived. When he tried to explain what had happened, he began laughing even harder.

When he was finally able to tell the nurse the whole story, he noticed that his pain was gone! He didn't need a shot at that time after all, and he didn't need to ask for another dose of pain medicine for another 90 minutes! (Source of story unknown.)

THE POWER OF CLEANLINESS

I have a friend who owns a car wash, and he's known to say that cars run a lot smoother when they're clean. The same could be said of our bodies and living spaces. People who keep their bodies and homes clean (and organized) are much more peaceful and efficient than those who have filthy homes and bodies.

It's true that everything looks and functions better when it's clean. That's because cleanliness is next to Godliness, and as children of God, we are hardwired to look and feel good (most comfortable) when all parts of us are clean and tidy. Think about it. Have you ever been embarrassed to let someone into your house because it was too clean? Or felt bad after showering and putting on freshly laundered clothes? Or worried about smelling or looking too good? And don't you always feel better after watching clean and uplifting movies than you do after watching a movie filled with foul language and smut?

Absolutely, being clean feels good, and being dirty makes us feel uncomfortable! Whether it is in our bodies, houses, yards, minds, or workplaces, filth and clutter always drag us down.

Feng Shui is an ancient Chinese art and science that uses colors and the arrangement of furniture and accessories to affect "energy flow" and to create harmony and balance. In Feng Shui, clutter represents stagnant and draining energy that can cause disturbances or dis-ease in both homes and in the health of the people who inhabit them. The energy of clutter clogs and interferes with the flow of healthy energy, which is why it's so important to regularly cleanse your inner body (blood and colon) and mind (do emotional release and meditate), as well as your body, clothes, and house.

Things that might need cleaning up are your clothes, body, mind, mouth, car, house, yard or garden, and/or environment around you.

THE POWER OF STRESS-RELIEF

The art of medicine consists of keeping the patient amused while nature heals the disease. Voltaire

When you continually feel overburdened and stressed, it creates an acidic system that cancer and other diseases thrive in. You don't have to be a stressed-out all the time; all you have to do is decide to handle things differently. To paraphrase Nelson Mandela, you, alone, are the captain of your own life. If you are ready to take control of your life and trade in stress for peace, here's how to do it:

• Get enough sleep—go to bed around 10:00 each night. To ensure peaceful sleep, make sure your room is pleasant, dark, quiet, and clutter-free, and unwind by doing something quiet and relaxing before bedtime. Sleep 7-8 hours a night.

• Get in the habit of getting up early and exercising first thing each day; then shower and dress before you greet the world. This will make you look and feel terrific.

• Bathe or shower daily. Brush your teeth at least two times a day, floss nightly, and keep your clothes, hair, and nails clean and well groomed. Everyone feels better when they practice good hygiene.

• Eat real and nutritious (unprocessed) food for breakfast. Avoid coffee, donuts, pastries, and other non-nutritious and harmful junk foods.

• Drink at least one half of your body weight in ounces of pure water each day. Stay away from soft drinks, energy drinks, processed juices (bottled or canned), sugar-free drinks (such as Crystal light), coffee drinks, sports drinks, and alcohol—all are very acidic, non-nutritious, and energy-depleting.

• Focus on one thing at a time. Do what's in your control and don't worry or think about anything else.

• If you can, turn off your cell phone most of the time. Only turn it on to make calls and check messages.

• Only check your e-mail once or twice a day. Delete messages that aren't pertinent if you don't have time to read them. Unsubscribe to newsletters and feeds that aren't serving you.

• Discipline yourself and finish up old tasks and projects before starting new ones.

• Give yourself permission to say no. Stop doing things out of obligation. Don't take on projects that aren't worth while. Do what makes your heart happy.

• Take charge of your money. Consolidate your debt and set up online checking. Set up automated payments and pay your bills online.

• Budget your spending and keep track of your money by writing down what you spend each day. It might surprise you how much you waste on frivolous things!

• Clean up and de-clutter. Go through your house, one room at a time, and get rid of all unnecessary items. Clean and organize what's left. Store sorted items in neatly labeled bins and containers.

• Keep your home and work areas clean. Do dishes, empty trash, and sweep, mop, dust, and vacuum regularly. When your environment is clean, you'll automatically feel lighter and more energetic.

• If you carry a purse, go through it often and get rid of what you don't need. Don't carry garbage and useless clutter around with you.

• Corral "car trash" by keeping a garbage bag in your car. Empty it daily or at least weekly.

• Instead of letting junk-mail stack up, get in the habit of shredding and recycling it as soon as it comes in.

• Copy important information such as bank and credit card numbers, social security numbers, driver's license numbers, and insurance information (and phone numbers to institutions), and keep the information in a safe and secure place so you'll know where it is if you need it.

• Keep touch with people you care about by making a list of addresses, phone numbers, and birthdays. Review it annually and keep it up to date. Send birthday cards to people you love.

• Buy and eat foods that will make you feel good, such as fresh seasonal produce and unprocessed grains and nuts. Avoid non-nutritious and processed foods.

• Create weekly meal plans, and only shop for groceries once a week.

• Keep a running list of items you need, and then plan shopping trips so that you can buy everything at once, while you're out, without backtracking.

• Keep a small notebook and pen with you at all times, and write things down as you think of them.

• Whenever you buy something new, go through your house and find something you no longer need and get rid of it. Recycle or donate used but still good items to a thrift store.

• Do laundry regularly, and keep your family's clothes organized and in good repair. Organize closets and drawers often. If you have too many clothes, get rid of what you don't wear. Only keep clothes that are versatile, practical, comfortable, and attractive. Only keep clothes that you love wearing—the ones that make you feel energetic and good about yourself.

• Refrain from buying clothing and accessories on impulse. Walk away from an item you like and think about it before you buy. Save money by only buying what you truly need or love.

• Avoid last minute crises by planning ahead and laying clothes out the night before, especially if you or your children have to leave early in the morning.

• Make lunches the night before—or at least do everything you can in advance.

• Schedule time to do things that you think are fun and rewarding. Make sure you're spending time doing things you like to do with people you enjoy being around.

• Be honest and full of integrity. Always be true to you!

• Be responsible. Do your fair share in life. Give more than you expect to get.

• Admit your mistakes. Whenever you realize that you've done something wrong, be accountable and quick to say "I'm sorry."

• Forgive yourself (and others) for being flawed. Give yourself (and others) a break when you (they) do something human. Don't waste energy being mad.

• Look for opportunities to serve others. It will help you forget your own problems.

• Ask for help when you need it. Say "I love you" and "thank you" a lot.

• Choose to be objective, positive, happy, and grateful. Count your blessings daily. Notice all the little things in your life that are good. Focus on what you have instead of what you want! Start a gratitude journal, and write in it often.

• Put yourself on a media diet. Limit Internet surfing and TV time, including watching movies and the news, to four hours or fewer per week.

• Create rewarding and uplifting rituals, and do them in the morning, afternoon, and/or evening—i.e., praying, meditating, reading inspiring literature (and scriptures), drinking herbal tea, writing in a journal, exercising, spending time with a child, developing a talent, working on crafts or a hobby, etc.

• Invest in your home, and make it an enjoyable and rewarding place to be. Save time and money by "staying in" for dates, meals, and entertainment.

• Spend time outside in the fresh air and sunshine. Try to take a walk each day. Don't forget to stop and smell the roses.

• Take regular "deep breathing" breaks. Relax, and simply focus on your breath.

• Find a massage therapist you like, and get a therapeutic massage regularly (like taking your car in for a tune-up).

• Avoid getting caught up in other people's drama. Create boundaries, and find new friends if you need to. Give family members and co-workers limits.

• Don't stress about doing everything on this list. Keep reading through it, and strive to improve daily.

• Throw out the word wrong and embrace the word different.

• Remember life is short and too precious to waste. Don't throw it away by being worried and stressed out; remember LIFE IS GOOD, and then relax and smile and thoroughly ENJOY one wonder-full day at a time!

The patient should be made to understand that he or she must take charge of his or her own life. Don't take your body to the doctor as if he were a repair shop. Quentin Regestein

IN SUMMATION

- CANCER (ETC.) CANNOT GROW IN AN ALKALINE BODY
Alkalize your system by eating mostly alkaline foods, drinking pure water, getting plenty of exercise, fresh air and sunshine, and reducing stress and being positive—this is the best type of preventive and curative medicine!

- PREVENTION IS THE VERY BEST MEDICINE!
An ounce of prevention is worth more than several pounds of cure. So starting today, begin taking steps towards living a healthier lifestyle. Rosemary and clove essential oil are known to prevent cancer—use these oils on a regular basis by applying them topically or by taking a few drops in a capsule.

- SUPPORT YOUR BODY (PREVENT DIS-EASE)
Incorporate as many natural "body building" treatments as you possibly can. For starters, make sure that you're eating a yeast-free diet, taking high quality supplements, using pure essential oils, and drinking close to 3/4 of your body weight in ounces of distilled or oxygenated water daily—the body requires one-half its body weight in ounces for maintenance, and three-quarters for healing.

   Do this even if you have been diagnosed with cancer and choose to do traditional medicine treatments such as chemotherapy and radiation. Your doctor may tell you not to, but keep in mind that it will not hurt you, and it will strengthen your body so that it can begin to self-heal! Many people who have taken Daily Supplements and used pure essential oils during chemotherapy and radiation have reported that they didn't experience much sickness or lose their hair.

- EARLY TREATMENT IS MOST EFFECTIVE!
If you suspect that you have cancer, don't delay in taking steps to treat it naturally. Sadly, I know many people who resisted alternative treatments until their doctor gave them no hope; and by then, it was too late for natural medicines to help them.

- DO ALL YOU CAN—THEN LIGHTEN UP & LET GO! Remember stress and worry can cause cancer and other diseases, but love, faith, prayer, and happiness have healing power. Don't forget to relax, B-R-E-A-T-H-E, and laugh every day!

- TRUST YOUR BODY
Do your best to treat your body right, and then BELIEVE IN THE SELF-HEALING MIRACLE THAT IS YOU!

Conventional cancer treatments are in place
as the law of the land because they pay, not heal, the best.
John Diamond, MD and Lee Cowden, MD

We kill with antibiotics and antiseptics,
and if our slaughter is ineffectual we use surgery to
expel the offending organ from our presence.
We destroy the body in order to save it.
Robert Svoboda

HELPFUL WEBSITES

• www.curezone.com = EDUCATION; vast amount of organized information about alternative medicines. This useful website is very easy to navigate.

• www.cancertutor.com = EDUCATION; lots of good information about cancer and alternative cancer treatments.

• www.naturalpedia.com = EDUCATION; lots of good information about cancer and other diseases and alternative treatments.

• www.mercola.com/forms/subscribe.htm = EDUCATION; signup page for Dr. Mercola's newsletter. Dr. Mercola is known as "the people's doctor" because he posts articles that contain "accurate and truthful" information about health.

• www.douglassreport.com = EDUCATION; Dr. Douglas' Daily Dose newsletter contains a variety of helpful and informative facts pertaining to health.

• www.naturalnews.com/Mike_Adams.html = EDUCATION; Mike Adams is journalist who covers scams. His Natural News newsletter reveals truth and offers natural solutions.

•www.naturessunshine.com/us/members/education/education1.aspx = EDUCATION; sign up for upcoming webinars and listen to webinars that cover a range of health-related subjects. Click on webinar archives.

- www.bestofrawfood.com = if you see the benefits of EATING RAW but are overwhelmed by the thought of it, this website will get you going.

- www.greensmoothiegirl.com = GREEN SMOOTHIE website; offers a lot of good solid information about nutrition and health. Make sure to take the free wellness quiz.

- www.greenpolkadotbox.com = online shopping portal where you can buy ORGANIC AND NATURAL PANTRY ITEMS at wholesale prices. This is a rewards–based buying group (like Costco), so you'll need to buy an annual membership. Tell your friends about the Green Polka-Dot Box, and when they sign up you'll earn points (free groceries) every time they shop. Shipping is free on orders over $150.00.

- www.eamega.com = where you can buy the "real-deal" AMEGA wand, pendent, and bracelet. Be sure to read testimonials.

- www.asea.com = where you can buy ASEA direct.

- www.iherbs.com = where you can buy Life's Basics PROTEIN POWDER for less. This plant-based vanilla protein is the best tasting (including whey) and healthiest protein powder I've ever tried. To get a big discount, open your own account, and then type "Life's Basics Plant Protein" in the search box. If you buy at least four containers at a time (15 servings each), you'll receive a discount plus free shipping. Get an additional discount by entering SUP832 in the "code box."

● www.planetsark.com = link to "Planet Sark." An imaginative and happy place to explore and hang out or to get cheered up and inspired. This is a great site to visit when you're feeling down!

The attitude you carry determines the direction your life will take. Believe in yourself, trust your instincts, and take responsibility for every decision you make. Anonymous

QUOTES WORTH PONDERING

♥ *Since cancer is caused primarily by environmental toxins and electro-magnetic pollution, the best way to prevent cancer is to minimize exposure to these influences. Eating organic food, using natural personal care and household cleaning products, and otherwise avoiding chemicals will help. For those toxins that can't be avoided, using antioxidant and hepatoprotective substances will minimize damage from chemicals.*
Steven Horne, RH (AHG), *The Comprehensive Guide to Nature's Sunshine Products*

♥ *(Regarding cancer) Avoid: refined grains and sugars, fried foods, and additives. Stay away from food colorings, coffee, tea, and cola drinks. Avoid meat, and eliminate salt-cured, salt-pickled, and smoked foods such as sausage, bacon, ham, smoked fish, bologna and hot dogs. A high-fat and meat diet can cause colon cancer. Fluoride in water and toothpaste is linked to bone cancer. Obesity increases the risk of colon cancer. Smoking causes lung and mouth cancer.* Louise Tenney, M.H., Nutritional Guide

♥ *Though not generally accepted, illness is fed by what we imbibe through the air and from the food and liquids we take. Conversely, as illness, including germs and viruses, cannot live in a clean environment, the solution is to abstain from food for a while and replace it with large amounts of clean water to purify the entire system.* Morris Krok

♥ *I believe that a toxic elimination system is the most common cause of ill health today, and the most dangerous. Fortunately it is also treatable.* Linda Berry, D.C.

♥ *74 percent of Americans are below daily RDA requirements for magnesium, 55 percent for iron, 68 percent calcium, 40 percent vitamin C, 33 percent B12, 80 percent B6, 33 percent B3, 3 percent B2, 45 percent B1, 50 percent vitamin A. From 25 to 50 percent of hospital patients suffer from protein calorie malnutrition. Pure malnutrition (cachexia) is responsible for at least 22 percent and up to 67 percent of all cancer deaths.*

Up to 80 percent of all cancer patients have reduced levels of serum albumin, which is a leading indicator of protein and calorie malnutrition. At least 20 percent of Americans are clinically malnourished, with 70 percent being sub-clinically malnourished, and the remaining "chosen few" 10 percent in good optimal health. Patrick Quillin, PhD

♥ *Pharmaceutical drugs are killing hundreds of thousands of people every year…In spite of that, they claim that two people were hurt with chaparral, so they have taken it off the market. And these claims aren't even substantiated.* Dr. Shulze

♥ *Homeopathy cures a larger percentage of cases than any other method of treatment and is beyond doubt safer and more economical and most complete medical science.* Mahatma Gandhi

♥ *In point of fact, fluoride causes more human cancer deaths, and causes it faster, than any other chemical.* Dean Burke, Former Chief Chemist Emeritus, U.S. National Cancer Institute

♥ *Since the human body tends to move in the direction of its expectations—plus or minus—it is important to know that attitudes of confidence and determination are no less a part of the treatment program than medical and science technology.* Norman Cousin

♥ *Pain (emotional, physical, mental) has a message. The information it has about our life can be remarkably specific, but it usually falls into one of two categories: "We would be more alive if we did more of this," and "Life would be more lovely if we did less of that." Once we get the pain's message, and follow its advice, the pain goes away.* Peter McWilliams

♥ *The competent physician, before he attempts to give medicine to the patient, makes himself acquainted not only with the disease, but also with the habits and constitution of the sick man.* Cicero

♥ *If people would take care of their body and cleanse their colon and intestines, their problems would be pretty much eliminated.*
Dr. George C. Crile

♥ *I truly believe the reason cancer rates and stress levels are rising is all the toxins we are absorbing through our food, air, and water.* Kevin Richardson

♥ *Everyone on this planet needs to be made aware that for several years now I have met and keep meeting people who no longer have AIDS, cancer, and almost any other disease you can think of, due to the continual and correct application of oxygen therapies.* Ed McCabe

♥ *In short, microwaves distort the molecular structure of the foods. They destroy much of the nutrients and cause many other problems with the immune system over a period of time. If you love your family, take the extra couple of minutes to heat the food up the right way.* Anthony Wayne and Lawrence Newell

♥ *As a people, we have become obsessed with health. There is something fundamentally, radically unhealthy about this. We do not seem to be seeking more exuberance in living as much as staving off failure; putting off dying. We have lost all confidence in the human body.* Lewis Thomas

♥ *A sad soul can kill you quicker than a germ.* John Steinbeck

♥ *Consult not your fears but your hopes and your dreams. Think not about your frustrations, but about your unfulfilled potential. Concern yourself not with what you tried and failed in, but what it is still possible for you to do.* Pope John XXIII

♥ *I say that habit's but a long practice, friend, and this becomes men's nature in the end.* Aristotle

♥ *From the bitterness of disease man learns the sweetness of health.* Catalan Proverb

♥ *You can complain because the roses have thorns, or you can rejoice because the thorns have roses.* Ziggy

♥ *People are like stained-glass windows. They sparkle and shine when the sun is out, but when the darkness sets in, their true beauty is revealed only if there is a light from within.* Elizabeth Kubler-Ross

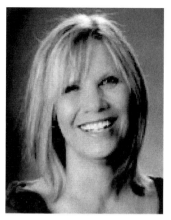

Connie Boucher (like touché) be-came unhappy with our current health-care system in the early nine-ties when she be¬came chronically ill and the prescription and over-the-counter medicines her doctor prescribed made her feel worse instead of better. After her doctor admitted that he'd tried everything he could think of and didn't have any solutions, she turned to natu-ral and alternative medicine for relief. When the herbs she'd been reluctant to take quickly healed a problematic sinus and bronchial infection, it piqued her interest and started her down a healer's path. Consequently, she became a massage thera-pist and then a wellness coach.

Connie's massage school¬ing, combined with a wide range of "natural healing" workshops and real-life experiences, have shaped her thinking and given her a unique perspective on life. She has a practical and open-minded way of viewing the world and solving her own problems, and she enthusiastically shares her stories, insights, and ever-expanding knowledge with others.

When it comes to being "right" about what she passionately teaches, Connie Boucher simply aligns herself with this quote by Mahatma Gandhi: "My aim is not to be consistent with any previous statement on a given question, but to be consistent with the truth as it may present itself on any given subject. The result is, I have grown from truth to truth."

Connie Boucher is the author of Super Simple Wellness, Wellness Made Simple, and Plain and Simple Flu Prevention.